CASE STUDIES IN UROLOGICAL CANCER

CASE STUDIES IN UROLOGICAL CANCER

Adrian N. Harnett

MBBS MRCP FRCR

Consultant in Clinical Oncology
Norfolk and Norwich University Hospital
Norwich, UK

Brian McGlynn

PostGradDip RGN

Specialist Nurse Urology Oncology
Ayr Hospital
Ayr, UK

Robert N. Meddings

MBChB BSc FRCS(Ed) FRCS (Urol) MD

Consultant Urologist
Ayr Hospital
Ayr, UK

With contributions from

Dr Stephen Cooper
Consultant Radiologist
Ayr Hospital
Ayr

Dr Bob Nairn
Consultant Pathologist
Crosshouse Hospital
Kilmarnock

GMM

LONDON ● SAN FRANCISCO

© 2003
Greenwich Medical Media Limited
137 Euston Road
London NW1 2AA

870 Market Street, Ste 720
San Francisco, CA 94102

ISBN 1 84110 138 9

First published 2003

A catalogue record for this book is available from the British Library.

Typeset by Phoenix Photosetting, Chatham, Kent

Printed in Italy by Giunti Industrie Grafiche

Distributed by Plymbridge Distributors Ltd and
in the USA by Jamco Distribution

www.greenwich-medical.co.uk

Contents

Foreword vii
Preface viii
Acknowledgements ix

SECTION 1: BLADDER 1

1. Immunotherapy in bladder cancer 3
2. Treatment for localised disease 7
3. Management of multiple tumours 9
4. Two primary urological tumours 13
5. Chemosensitive bladder carcinoma 17
6. Renal failure and chemotherapy 21

SECTION 2: PROSTATE 25

1. A prostate cancer dilemma 27
2. Treatment for early stage disease 31
3. Metastatic disease or not? 35
4. Bone scan for low risk disease? 37
5. Multiple urological tumours 41
6. Solitary bone metastasis 45
7. Spinal cord compression 51
8. Unusual sites of metastatic disease 55
9. Prostate cancer and liver metastases 59
10. Bone marrow infiltration 65

SECTION 3: KIDNEY 71

1. Adapting treatment for an unusual situation 73
2. Management of a complex renal cyst 77
3. The equivocal renal carcinoma 81
4. Surveillance of the upper urinary tract 85
5. Immunotherapy sensitive renal carcinoma 91
6. The role of surgery 97
7. Metastatic disease, unknown primary 101

SECTION 4: PENIS 107

1. *In situ* disease 109
2. The unusual location 111
3. The unusual tumour 113
4. Primary or metastatic? 115

SECTION 5: TESTIS 119

1. The common tumour 121
2. The unusual tumour 123
3. Testicular pain from a rare tumour 125
4. The extratesticular tumour 127
5. Metastatic teratoma at presentation 131
6. Metastatic seminoma at presentation 135

APPENDICES 137

Appendix   I   Selected trials 139
Appendix   II   Drugs used in urological cancer
                        treatment 141
Appendix III   Hormone therapy guideline for prostate
                        cancer 143
Appendix IV   PSA 145
Appendix   V   TNM staging 147
Appendix VI   Gleason score 149
Appendix VII   Recommended reading 151

INDEX 153

Foreword

The term 'Urological Cancer' encompasses five tumour types, extremely diverse in their incidence, presentation, and management. Adeno-carcinoma of the prostate is one of the commonest male malignancies, while squamous carcinoma of the penis is among the rarest. Tumours of the testis occur predominantly in young men while bladder and prostate cancer are essentially (but not entirely) diseases of old age. Advances in oncology have rendered testicular cancer, even when it presents with metastatic disease, a curable condition with long-term disease-free survival rates in excess of 90%, while the mortality from bladder cancer has not changed significantly. Prostate cancer presents the greatest dilemma – despite being one of the commonest causes of cancer mortality in men, many men with the disease do not die from it. The introduction of PSA testing and transrectal ultrasound guided biopsy have made it far easier to diagnose the condition in many more men and at an earlier stage. Does this mean that we can now cure men who in the past presented with advanced disease, or are we subjecting many men with insignificant disease to unnecessary aggressive treatment? Certainly we should reserve judgement as to how these advances will affect mortality in the long term, and all would agree that many men with prostate cancer do not need immediate treatment, surely an almost unique situation in oncology.

The many dilemmas in the diagnosis and management of urological cancer are illustrated by the cases described in this book. The optimum management of most forms of urological cancer requires a multi-disci-plinary approach, and this is reflected in the authorship. The team at The Ayr Hospital have shown that even complex treatment of the majority of these cancers can be managed in District General Hospitals where there is a sufficient population basis and when local expertise is available to provide the specialist care that is required. I consider the inclusion of a Nurse Specialist among the authors to be particularly significant. In the management of urological cancers, the role of the specialist nurse in coordination, counselling and support during treatment is invaluable and the team at The Ayr Hospital have been in the forefront of developing this type of service. I commend them for their contribution and their book to its readers.

Professor David Kirk
Department of Urology
Gartnavel General Hospital
Glasgow
January 2003

Preface

The first book in the *Case Studies* series was published almost a year ago. It covered breast cancer and was illustrated by 'real cases' from diagnostic dilemmas right through to palliative care issues. It was written in a format that put the reader in the clinician's shoes and focused on how management decisions are often not clear cut and sometimes frankly controversial. What would the reader do? Often, what is seen in clinical practice cannot be found in textbooks and it is a challenge to know what is right. It is then that the value of experience and the wisdom of the multi-disciplinary team come into effect.

For the second book we move on to urological cancer but have largely kept the same popular format. The authors represent an urologist, urology specialist nurse and an oncologist, all vital members of the multi-disciplinary team. There are five sections covering the different tumour sites of bladder, prostate, kidney, penis and testis. Obviously, the incidence of the first two tumour sites is far more frequent than the last two but we have tried to achieve a reasonable balance of cases across the groups. As with the breast cancer book, cases are presented in each section starting with early stage disease and progressing through to treatment-sensitive metastatic disease and then to aggressive and refractory advanced disease. Again, the text for the illustrations has been kept to a minimum so that you can answer the questions posed and decide what abnormalities are being shown without being pre-empted. You may even wish to look at the illustrations first before reading *any* of the text.

Some of the case histories may appear incomplete. This is either because their clinical history continues or because only the most interesting part of their care has been presented. However, they are all patients who have been managed through the Ayrshire Urological Oncology Group and who have trusted us with their care. Very few, (if any), of the details have been changed. It should be borne in mind that some patients were initially treated quite a while ago and so their management now could be significantly different.

In writing this second book we hope, like us, that it will prompt you to think about new ways to care for your patients, who continue to impress us by the way they cope with the challenges of life. In many respects they are our teachers.

Adrian Harnett
Brian McGlynn
Bob Meddings
January 2003

Acknowledgements

We are grateful to the many people who have been involved in making this book possible. We particularly thank colleagues in the multidisciplinary teams, namely urologists, specialist nurses, clinic and ward nurses, radiologists, pathologists and palliative care physicians.

In particular, we would like to thank our surgical colleagues for the advice and support, namely Mr Gerry Watson, Mr Murat Gurun, Mr Nils Al-Saffar, Professor David Kirk and Mr Graham Hollins, some of whom have referred cases and all of whom have been involved directly in their management. The assistance of Dr Stephen Cooper, Consultant Radiologist and Dr Bob Nairn, Consultant Pathologist, has been particularly invaluable. Dr Pauline Vosylius, Consultant Haematologist and Dr Robin Reid, Consultant Pathologist, have also given advice and assisted in the management of some of the patients.

Caroline Eadie and other staff from medical illustration at the Western Infirmary and Crosshouse Hospitals have processed the figures. Margaret Fierney, pharmacist in Ayr Hospital, has given advice on prescribing, particularly with Appendix III. Ailsa Griffen has again given secretarial support and coordinated the project with us.

Finally, it has been a pleasure to have the assistance of AstraZeneca again, particularly Tim Sherwell, and Gavin Smith from Greenwich Medical Media. This book is an illustration of a urological multidisciplinary team recounting examples of patients who have come under our care. They are the biggest contributors and it is to them that we express our most thanks.

ANH
BMcG
RNM

SECTION 1: BLADDER

Case 1   Immunotherapy in bladder cancer   3
Case 2   Treatment for localised disease   7
Case 3   Management of multiple tumours   9
Case 4   Two primary urological tumours   13
Case 5   Chemosensitive bladder carcinoma   17
Case 6   Renal failure and chemotherapy   21

Case 1: Immunotherapy in bladder cancer

A 45-year-old man presented with a history of several months of intermittent difficulty in voiding, urinary frequency and dysuria. A diagnosis of possible prostatitis or bladder outflow obstruction was made. An IVU and PSA were normal. Flexible cystoscopy revealed a ring like hypertrophied bladder neck with some erythematous areas in the bladder. At first the patient was treated as having benign disease; however, he continued to complain of suprapubic pain and irritative lower urinary symptoms over the next two months.

What treatment recommendations would you make?

On account of persistent irritative symptoms and pain, the patient underwent a GA cystoscopy which again showed an erythematous area over the bladder trigone and extending on the right lateral wall above the right ureteric orifice. Biopsy of this area revealed *in situ* disease (**Figure 1.1.1**).

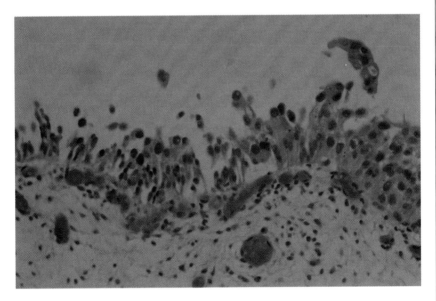

Figure 1.1.1   Carcinoma *in situ*, H&E × 64

What further treatment would you recommend?

A further GA procedure and resection of the whole erythematous area was performed which confirmed *in situ* disease again. He was commenced on intravesical BCG, receiving six instillations over a two-month period. After this therapy, a further cystoscopy was carried out, which showed an excellent response with marked regression of the changes in the bladder. There was general erythema of the mucosa and further biopsies were taken which showed evidence of granulomata, (**Figure 1.1.2**) but no evidence of *in situ* or invasive tumour. At the completion of BCG therapy, his urinary symptoms had completely resolved.

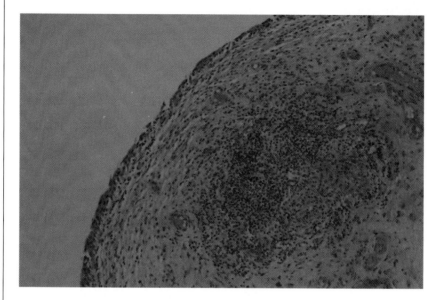

Figure 1.1.2   Bladder mucosa with BCG granuloma, H&E × 32

There is some debate about whether, or indeed how, maintenance immunotherapy should be given. In our unit, maintenance is based on a single instillation of intravesical BCG every six months. He also received oral Trimethoprim when having the BCG, as this was previously associated with infection.

He continues on maintenance immunotherapy and has regular check cystoscopies, none of which have shown recurrence of the *in situ* disease. Over 5 years from initial presentation, bladder biopsies show only chronic inflammation, while the transitional epithelium shows mild reactive changes but no evidence of dysplasia or malignancy (**Figure 1.1.3**). Some centres favour using the more conventional three instillations rather than one.

This case demonstrates the importance of biopsying patients who

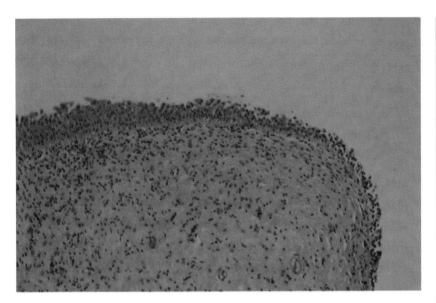

Figure 1.1.3 Normal urothelium with mild inflammation, H&E × 32

have significant irritative symptoms and bladder pain. This also indicates the excellent response that can occur with conservative management of carcinoma *in situ*, particularly when there is not a general field change but when there is a patch of confined disease.

Case 2: Treatment for localised disease

A 72-year-old retired golfer presented having had a couple of black-outs. Blood tests carried out by her GP showed an elevated creatinine level. She had an ultrasound scan, which revealed a lesion in the bladder. There were no urinary symptoms.

How would you manage this patient?

Further renal function was satisfactory and so cystourethroscopy was performed. This revealed a tumour on the left lateral wall of the bladder, which was partially resected. Neither ureteric orifice was involved. Pathology revealed a grade 3 transitional cell carcinoma invading muscle (**Figure 1.2.1**).

Bladder carcinoma most frequently presents with painless haematuria, so this was a slightly unusual presentation. A CT scan of the abdomen and pelvis was carried out (**Figure 1.2.2**).

What do these figures show?

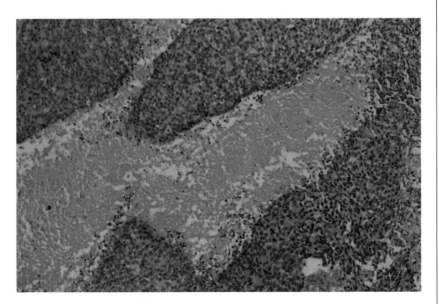

Figure 1.2.1 Solid transitional cell carcinoma grade 3 with necrosis, H&E × 32

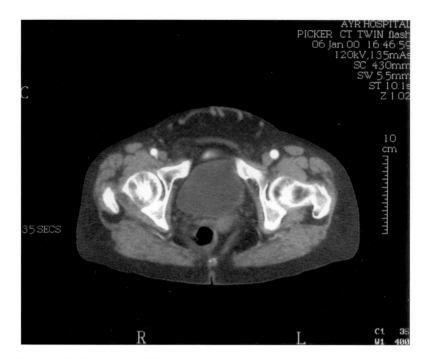

AYR HOSPITAL
PICKER CT TWIN flash
06 Jan 00 16:46:59
120kV,135mAs
SC 430mm
SW 5.5mm
ST 10.1s
Z 1.02

10
cm

35 SECS

R   L

C1 35
W1 400

Figure 1.2.2 CT scan of pelvis

The CT scan showed some thickening on the left lateral wall of the bladder in keeping with tumour. No other abnormality was demonstrated. As she had high-grade disease involving muscle she required definitive treatment with either surgery (radical cystectomy) or a course of external beam radiotherapy. Surgery is more frequently performed in younger patients. In patients over 65, treatment is more often given by radical radiotherapy. She was planned for a course of radiotherapy, receiving 52.4 Gy in 20 fractions over four weeks, using a 4-field megavoltage isocentric technique. She tolerated treatment well. She developed a mild perineal reaction and radiation cystitis, which rapidly settled.

Following radiotherapy, she has remained well and leads a very active life. She has no symptoms from her urinary tract and after three years follow up, the most recent check cystoscopy showed no evidence of recurrence, just telangiectasis in the bladder as a result of radiotherapy. She remains very well.

Case 3: Management of multiple tumours

A 48-year-old nurse presented nine years ago with painless haematuria. She was otherwise well and at cystoscopy there was a solitary papillary bladder tumour, which was completely resected. The upper urinary tract showed no abnormality. Pathological examination (**Figure 1.3.1**) confirmed low-grade papillary transitional cell carcinoma, (pTa G1).

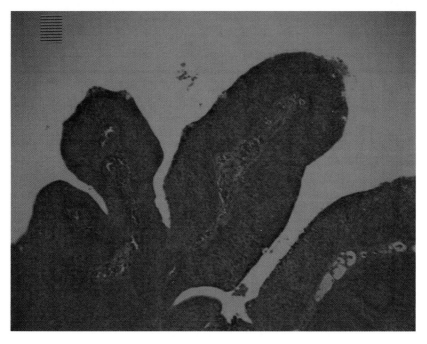

Figure 1.3.1   Original tumour biopsy, low grade transitional cell carcinoma, H&E scale 0.1 mm (top left)

What management would you recommend?

It was decided to institute a policy of cystoscopic surveillance. If she were to be treated now, she would be managed more actively, probably using intravesical chemotherapy after initial tumour resection. The patient was followed up and cystoscopy three months later showed recurrent papillary disease, which was treated with diathermy. At each subsequent cystoscopy, there were either single or multiple bladder tumour recurrences, all of which were managed with diathermy or resection. Three years later she had a course of intravesical Epirubicin and a further two years later, Mitomycin. Despite these interventions, she still had repeated recurrences. Pathology throughout showed the disease was always superficial and low grade, (pTa G1 disease). There was no evidence of subepithelial invasion. Six years after her initial diagnosis, she was treated with intravesical BCG and responded. Maintenance treatment was given on a six-monthly basis, comprising single instillations of BCG.

How should this patient be managed at this stage?

Should cystectomy be performed?

Six years after the original diagnosis she still developed recurrent multifocal superficial transitional cell cancer, which was low grade and with no evidence of invasion (**Figure 1.3.2**). Radiotherapy is not usually employed with superficial tumours but the disease has not been controlled by intravesical chemotherapy. Although there has been some improvement with intravesical BCG, recurrence still occurs. She remains asymptomatic and is only troubled by her attendances for cystoscopy.

Radical cystectomy in the absence of invasion and for low-grade disease would appear a little too aggressive but she was at risk of developing further tumours in the renal tract. She therefore continued for the next three and a half years with three-monthly checks and regular cystodiathermy.

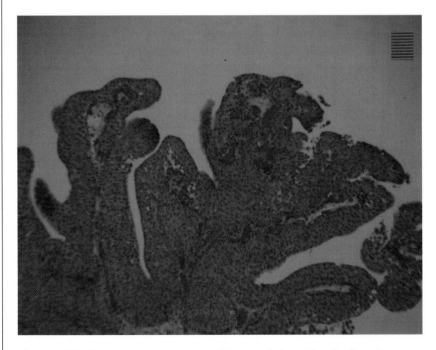

Figures 1.3.2 Most recent occurrence, still low grade transitional cell carcinoma, H&E scale 0.1 mm (top right)

Radiological surveillance with intravenous urography was repeated at four years and eight years following diagnosis. At eight years she developed a superficial transitional cell tumour of the left renal pelvis. This was confirmed on retrograde examination and ureteroscopy.

Is radical surgery now required?

The presence of disease in the upper tracts would perhaps warrant radical surgery with a left nephro-ureterectomy. If this line of radical management is followed then, logically, radical cystectomy should be done. This would leave a solitary kidney only, which also has the risk of developing transitional cell cancer. An alternative strategy is conservative management with organ preservation, endoscopic treatment of recurrence and further surveillance.

The options were discussed with the patient, (including cystectomy and orthotopic reconstruction) and she preferred the less interventional course. She was referred for laser ablation of the superficial transitional cell cancer using a flexible ureteroscope. This was successfully achieved and recent radiology and ureteroscopy have shown no evidence of recurrent superficial disease in the left upper tract. She remains well and with a good quality of life, which is only interrupted for short periods following her regular cystoscopic interventions.

Comment

On balance, this patient has a greater chance of significant morbidity and complications due to surgery than she does from the organ conservation option. The likelihood is that these superficial transitional tumors may never progress and be life threatening. The difficulty in monitoring and treating the upper tracts has eased with the improvement of flexible ureteroscopy and the availability of laser tumour ablation. Clearly, close monitoring of her upper tracts is going to be important in her follow up. Now, almost ten years following her diagnosis, there has been no significant change in the histological grade of the tumours and it appears unlikely that she will develop life-threatening disease.

Case 4: Two primary urological tumours

A 65-year-old heating engineer presented with symptoms of frequency, nocturia and urgency. Rectal examination revealed a hard right lobe of prostate and biopsies showed well-differentiated adeno-carcinoma. The PSA was elevated at 13.

What investigations and treatment would you recommend?

Routine staging investigations including a bone and MRI scan confirmed localised prostate cancer. In view of his age and good health, he was offered radical treatment, either with surgery or external radio-therapy. With similar results achieved by either radical therapy, patients should be involved in the choice of treatment. The patient chose the surgical option and this was carried out.

He recovered well following surgery. Pathology showed prostatic adenocarcinoma (**Figure 1.4.1**) with evidence of marked perineural involvement posteriorly and there was tumour microscopically at the posterior margin. He suffered very few urinary side effects post-operatively. He was completely continent within three months following

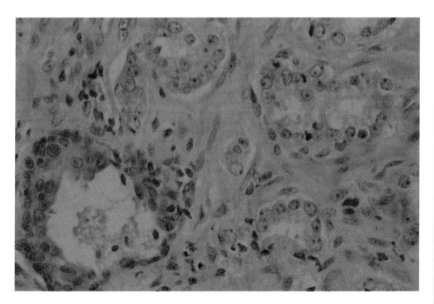

Figure 1.4.1 Radical prostatectomy with infiltrating prostatic adenocarcinoma, H&E × 128

surgery and was prescribed an anti-cholinergic which he later discontinued as his symptoms had improved significantly. He had erectile dysfunction, but declined any further intervention for this problem. The PSA dropped to an undetectable level immediately following operation and has remained on or around this level for more than five years.

At a routine clinic review he complained of irritable bladder symptoms along with a single episode of haematuria. An MSSU showed red blood cells only and culture revealed no growth. A flexible cystoscopy revealed a superficial bladder tumour along the left lateral wall of the bladder with a few smaller tumours scattered just inside the bladder neck. The patient had resection of tumour, and pathology confirmed superficial but high-grade disease, (pT1 G3).

How should this patient be managed?

A staging CT scan of the abdomen and pelvis did not demonstrate any bladder tumour, perivesical extension or lymphadenopathy. An incidental finding on the CT scan of the chest was asbestos-related lung disease with calcified pleural plaques (**Figure 1.4.2**) due to his previous occupation. The patient had no respiratory symptoms.

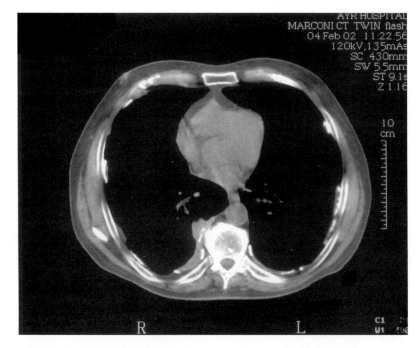

Figure 1.4.2 CT scan of the chest shows calcified pleural plaques typical of asbestos-related lung disease. A smaller area of focal pleural thickening in the right paravertebral area was followed up to confirm that it was related to previous asbestos exposure rather than being due to a pleural metastatic deposit.

The options for management were radical surgery, intravesical chemotherapy or immunotherapy. Initially, he was treated with intravesical Mitomycin and on follow-up there was little response and he still had pT1 G3 disease with associated carcinoma *in situ*. This was then treated with intravesical BCG again with little response, and when re-biopsied, there was still pT1 G3 disease and *in situ* carcinoma (**Figure 1.4.3**).

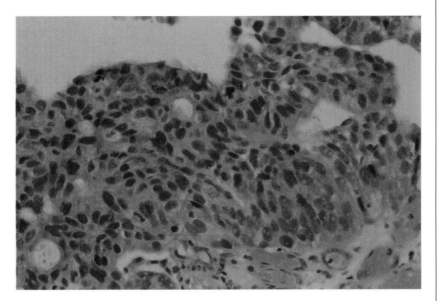

Figure 1.4.3   Grade 3 papillary transitional cell carcinoma, H&E × 64

How would you further manage this patient?

The patient, who had previously undergone radical surgery with curative intent for an early prostate cancer, has now developed a transitional cell tumour, which has not responded to intravesical chemotherapy or immunotherapy. He is a well-motivated patient who is now 70 years of age and in view of his excellent general health, he required radical definitive treatment and opted for cystectomy. Interestingly, the surgical option of an orthotopic reconstruction was intended, but a standard ileal conduit was constructed due to peri-urethral scarring preventing adequate reconstruction. The patient remains well over one year later.

Case 5: Chemosensitive bladder carcinoma

A 63-year-old butcher presented with intermittent haematuria. He was found to have a solid tumour on the right side of the bladder, which was completely resected. The bladder was generally erythematous. Four quadrant biopsies were also taken. Histology revealed a superficial papillary grade 3 transitional cell carcinoma (**Figure 1.5.1**). There was no muscle infiltration. There was some dysplasia in the random bladder biopsies. Six weeks later, a further cystoscopy revealed recurrence and extension of the right-sided disease onto the roof of the bladder by high-grade transitional carcinoma which was invading muscle.

How should this patient be managed?

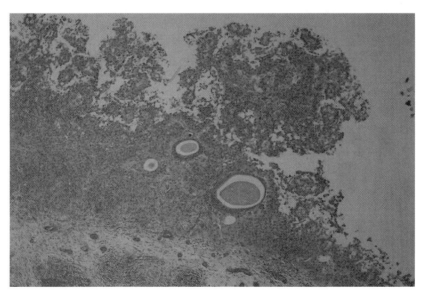

Figure 1.5.1 Papillary transitional cell carcinoma of the bladder with superficial infiltration, H&E × 12.8

This man appeared to have aggressive disease, as shown by quite significant changes at cystoscopy over a very short interval of time. Also, histology revealed a poorly differentiated tumour. A CT scan was therefore performed (**Figure 1.5.2**). This showed extensive bladder wall thickening involving the whole of the right lateral wall and most of the anterior surface of the bladder. There was marked extravesical extension, although the seminal vesicles and prostate did not appear to be involved. There were enlarged pelvic lymph nodes, particularly on the right hand side. The patient continued to complain of haematuria.

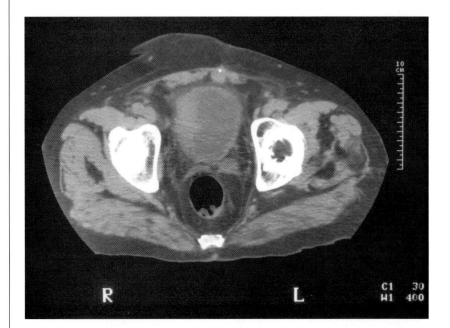

Figure 1.5.2

What treatment options are available?

He obviously had an inoperable tumour. One treatment option would have been palliative radiotherapy, which may cause resolution of the haematuria. An appropriate dose is a single fraction using parallel-opposed fields or a short fractionated course, such as 20 Gy in five fractions over one week. However, the patient had good health, continued to work and was keen to be actively managed. Renal function was satisfactory and he therefore received chemotherapy with Cisplatin, Methotrexate and Vinblastine. He tolerated the first three courses of chemotherapy well. A repeat CT scan showed resolution of the lymphadenopathy and marked regression of the bladder wall thickening indicating an excellent response to chemotherapy. He received a further two courses of chemotherapy but the doses had to be reduced due to deteriorating renal function. He was quite unwell at the time, had symptoms suggestive of a gastrointestinal bleed and was commenced on Ranitidine. He was given blood transfusion support and gradually recovered.

At this point he did not want any further treatment and was put on follow-up. He had intermittent haematuria.

He remained well for a year but was then admitted due to anaemia, with two recent episodes of haematemesis. He had a previous history of a perforated gastric ulcer and excessive alcohol intake. Upper gastrointestinal endoscopy was performed, which showed inflammatory changes in the antrum of the stomach and duodenal bulb. He was discharged on Lisinopril and Lansoprazole. He had no evidence of *Helicobacter*.

A few months later he had marked haematuria. Cystourethroscopy revealed a tumour, again on the right side of the bladder, which was fairly localised.

Discuss his management

He had had an excellent response to chemotherapy and received a palliative course of radiotherapy, receiving 20 Gy in five fractions with parallel-opposed fields.

He was reviewed regularly in the clinic and 18 months later remained well. He has had a most impressive response to both chemotherapy and, more recently, radiotherapy, and it was therefore decided to perform a further check cystoscopy. There was recurrence with superficial papillary lesions below the right ureteric orifice and the area looked oedematous. Histology revealed just transitional carcinoma *in situ* with no evidence of invasive disease.

What further management would you recommend?

This patient originally presented with advanced bladder carcinoma. At cystoscopy he had only superficial disease and therefore one could make an argument for not performing any active management at this stage. It was decided to arrange a further CT scan, which showed no lymphadenopathy and no abnormality in the bladder apart from thickening of the bladder wall. The patient was feeling very well and was happy to have active treatment and so intravesical BCG instillation was carried out. He received six-weekly instillations and then a repeat cystoscopy was peformed, which showed a few erythematous areas in the bladder but no obvious tumour. Biopsies showed chronic inflammation only and no evidence of any residual tumour.

The patient was admitted as a medical emergency six months later and the diagnosis of a brain stem infarct was made. CT scan of the brain did not show any evidence of brain metastases. He died five days after admission.

Comment

This patient demonstrated an excellent and unusual response to both chemotherapy and later radiotherapy having presented with metastatic bladder carcinoma. In a way, the impressive response made later management decisions more difficult. The pathology and radiology were reviewed and confirmed during his subsequent management.

The patient therefore lived for over five years after presenting with locally extensive pelvic disease and died due to an apparently separate vascular event.

Case 6: Renal failure and chemotherapy

A 58-year-old nursing tutor presented with a one-year history of increased frequency of micturition and occasional haematuria. He had lost a stone in weight over the last two months. He complained of fatigue but had no pain. Blood tests revealed a urea of 39.4 and serum creatinine of 655.

How would you manage this patient?

He was admitted for further management as he was in renal failure. Ultrasound showed bilateral hydronephrosis, (**Figure 1.6.1 & Figure 1.6.2**) and a 2–3 cm soft tissue thickening at the bladder base involving both ureteric orifices. It was presumed that he had a bladder carcinoma obstructing both ureters and went on to have bilateral nephrostomies inserted. Clinical examination also revealed left supraclavicular lymphadenopathy. CT scan was performed (**Figure 1.6.3 & Figure 1.6.4**).

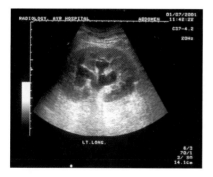

Figure 1.6.1
Ultrasound scans of kidneys

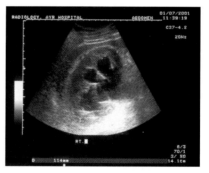

Figure 1.6.2

What does this show?

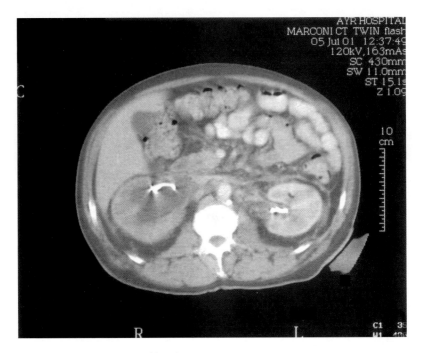

Figure 1.6.3 CT scan at renal level

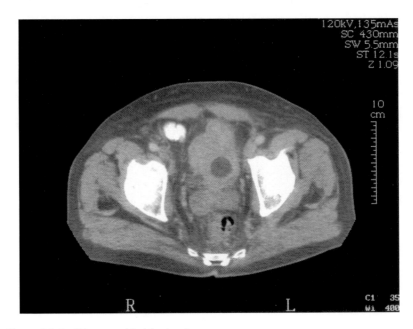

Figure 1.6.4 CT scan at bladder level

The renal function improved so that cystoscopy could be performed. This showed that the bladder was full of tumour and was reduced to a small capacity. Pathology revealed a poorly differentiated transitional cell carcinoma, (**Figure 1.6.5**). The CT scan confirmed the extensive bladder carcinoma with bilateral inguinal lymphadenopathy and para-aortic lymphadenopathy. Nephrostomies can be seen in the renal pelves. He also had subcutaneous deposits in the left supraclavicular fossa and left inguinal region.

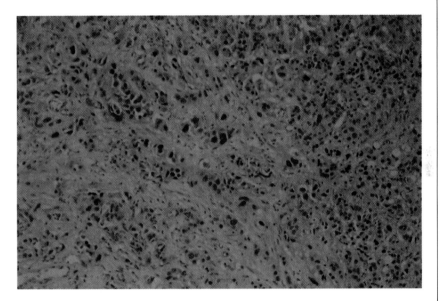

Figure 1.6.5   Infiltrating grade 3 TCC, H&E × 64

What management would you propose?

Antegrade stenting was performed and the bilateral nephrostomies removed. He was very keen to have active therapy but understood that he had widespread metastatic and locally advanced carcinoma of the bladder. Although renal function had improved, his urea remained raised at 13 and calculated creatinine clearance was 45. In view of the very compromised renal function, he had a very modified dose of Cisplatin, Methotrexate and Vinblastine (CMV). After the first course of treatment, there was considerable regression of the soft tissue disease in both inguinal and supraclavicular regions. He also felt a lot better and put on weight. Therefore, chemotherapy was continued for five courses. Renal function remained stable throughout.

Within a couple of weeks of stopping chemotherapy, the soft tissue disease progressed and the patient did not feel so well. He therefore received another three courses of modified CMV chemotherapy with response. However, his ultimate prognosis remained very poor.

It is unusual to use Cisplatin-based chemotherapy with severe renal dysfunction. However, the treatment options were very limited, the patient was symptomatic and he very much wished to have active management. As a result of his occupation, he was very well informed. He tolerated the chemotherapy well and understood the risk of receiving it under these conditions. He actually managed to continue as a lecturer in nursing throughout his chemotherapy.

SECTION 2: PROSTATE

Case 1   A prostate cancer dilemma?   27
Case 2   Treatment for early stage disease   31
Case 3   Metastatic disease or not?   35
Case 4   Bone scan for low risk disease?   37
Case 5   Multiple urological tumours   41
Case 6   Solitary bone metastasis   45
Case 7   Spinal cord compression   51
Case 8   Unusual sites of metastatic disease   55
Case 9   Prostate cancer and liver metastases?   59
Case 10   Bone marrow infiltration   65

Case 1: A prostate cancer dilemma?

A 45-year-old gentleman presented with haematuria, fever and generally feeling unwell. He was treated by his GP with antibiotics but continued to have marked urinary frequency with severe urgency and intermittent haematuria over a six-month period. A rectal examination revealed a clinically benign but mildly tender prostate gland and abdominal examination revealed no abnormality.

How would you manage this patient?

A clinical diagnosis of prostatitis was made. The PSA was 4.1. Routine radiological investigations were normal, as was flexible cystoscopy. Initially, the patient was treated conservatively by the use of antibiotics and anti-inflammatories. There had been no evidence of infection on urine culture on several occasions. He had a mildly impaired flow pattern and therefore was started on α-blockade (Alfuzosin). He had some improvement of his symptoms and his haematuria settled, but he still had urinary frequency and felt unwell. The PSA remained slighty elevated at 4.2.

Would it be reasonable to proceed with transrectal ultrasound and biopsy or would that make his presumed diagnosis of prostatitis worse?

The absence of a conclusive diagnosis, the possibility of an underlying malignancy and a consistently elevated PSA in a 45-year-old man were strong indications for prostate biopsy. This was carried out. The risks of severe septic complications from the procedure are less than 1%. The gland volume was 33 ml with some calcification in the gland but no other obvious abnormality. Sextant biopsies were performed and prostate biopsies in one of the cores showed a focal group of glands, which were highly suspicious of malignancy (**Figure 2.1.1**). Further biopsies were advised.

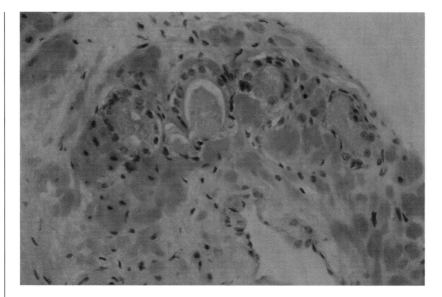

Figure 2.1.1 Four malignant glands in a prostate core biopsy, H&E × 64

How would you proceed?

The patient was told of the suspicion of malignancy on the biopsies. A further set of ultrasound-guided biopsies was taken under general anaesthetic and all 12 biopsies were benign. They were repeated four months later with the same result.

How would you manage this patient?

A further pathologist reviewed all of the biopsies. She agreed that the first biopsies had features of carcinoma and confirmed that malignancy was not present in any other biopsies. Occasionally, the pathologist may have difficulty in interpretation and making a diagnosis of cancer on needle biopsies of the prostate and so it is important they are reviewed in contentious cases.

The patient had a localised prostate cancer but with only a minute focus of disease. Radical treatment in the form of surgery or radio-therapy, (and possibly brachytherapy), could have been be given. An alternative strategy would have been to carry out observation and not give any initial active treatment, as he had an intraepithelial focus of malignancy that may never progress to invasive carcinoma. There was even the possibility of spontaneous tumour regression in this situation. Indeed, he had a demanding job, was fit and well and did not want radical surgery or radiotherapy. He therefore opted for a watch-and-wait policy. The PSA came down to 1.4 without treatment and his symptoms over the next 9–12 months gradually resolved. With such a small focus of disease and a PSA returning to normal limits, the implications and consequences of radical treatment must be very carefully considered.

The patient, with his wife, agreed to a conservative policy, involving follow-up rectal examinations and PSA monitoring. If the PSA started to rise again, further prostate biopsies would be needed.

Case 2: Treatment for early stage disease

This very well 65-year-old man presented with lower urinary symptoms and an elevated PSA of 13. On rectal examination, the prostate was hard on the left side and felt nodular. Transrectal ultrasound biopsies confirmed the diagnosis of a Gleason 6 adenocarcinoma of the prostate with perineural and vascular channel involvement. Full staging with an MRI scan of the pelvis confirmed localised disease with no extension into the peri-prostatic venous plexus, pelvic side-wall, seminal vesicles or rectum, (**Figure 2.2.1**). A bone scan was normal.

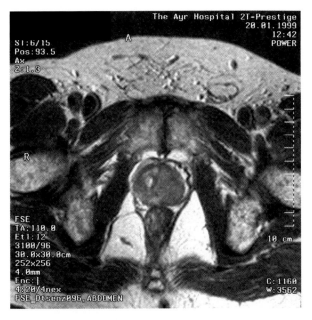

Figure 2.2.1 The prostatic tumour cannot be clearly identified on the MRI scan. A focus of high signal on the right side of the gland is believed to be due to a small focus of haemorrhage within the gland following recent biopsies.

How would you manage this patient?

According to Partin's tables, the possibility of this man having organ-confined disease with a Gleason score of 6 and PSA of 13 is 38%. However, it was felt reasonable to offer radical treament and the patient's preference was for surgery. A programme of laparoscopic radical prostatectomy had been commenced and this was discussed with the patient, who wished to pursue this option. He was started on Casodex monotherapy and after three months he underwent a laparoscopic radical prostatectomy. There was some urine leakage from the abdominal drain during the first six days but this then settled. Subsequent pathology showed that there was disease present at the resection margins both anteriorly and posteriorly, and also disease within the peri-urethral tissue blocks. The patient was admitted two weeks post-operatively with haematuria and profuse leakage of urine per rectum. At no time was he unwell or septic.

How would you manage this complication?

The patient had a cystogram (**Figure 2.2.2**), which showed a leakage at the level of the bladder neck and urethral anastomosis with a long fistula tract entering into the upper rectum. This was probably a late manifestation of rectal injury by diathermy at the time of surgery.

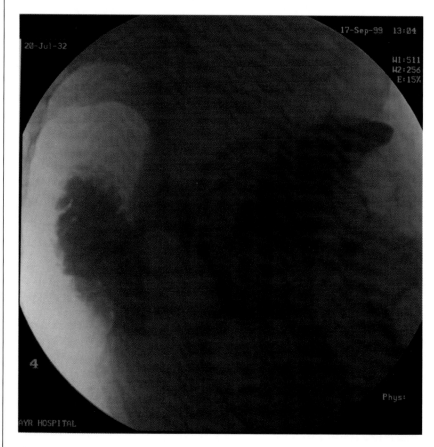

Figure 2.2.2 Cystogram

How should this gentleman's urethro-rectal fistula be managed?

The usual surgical management of a case of this nature would be to perform a defunctioning colostomy and, at the same time, repair the anastomosis between the urethra and the bladder neck. At no time was the patient septic nor did the patient wish to have open surgery. So far he had radical surgery for localised prostate cancer and had avoided an abdominal wound.

It was planned to manage the patient by diverting the urine through large 8 French ureteric catheters and a urethral catheter in order to see if the fistula would close spontaneously. At cystoscopy the obvious dehiscence of the anastomosis between the bladder neck and urethra on the right side was apparent. Also, on this side, it was not possible to see the opening of the right ureter. As a result, an 8 French catheter was passed up the left ureter only. An antegrade study delineated the right system and a nephrostomy tube was inserted. At a further cystoscopy, a guide wire was passed into the bladder through the nephrostomy and an 8 French ureteric catheter inserted into the right ureter along the guide wire. Following the successful placement of two ureteric catheters and a urethral catheter, the leakage from the rectum gradually resolved over a period of 48 hours. The patient was left with an indwelling Silastic urethral catheter with two ureteric catheters running adjacent to this, (**Figure 2.2.3**).

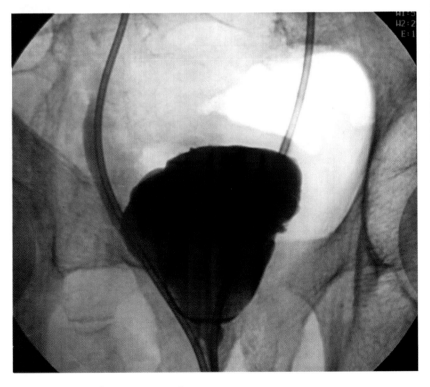

Figure 2.2.3 Further contrast study

The patient was very co-operative and very well motivated and managed for a total of 82 days with this arrangement of urinary drainage. There was no further leakage of the urine from the rectum. Subsequent cystogram showed the fistula tract had closed spontaneously (**Figure 2.2.4**) and the catheters were removed. The patient was left with a little stress wetting. Three years following his original surgery he does not require the use of any continence aids, he is able to achieve erections by the use of Sildenafil and the last PSA level measurement was 0.2. There is no palpable disease.

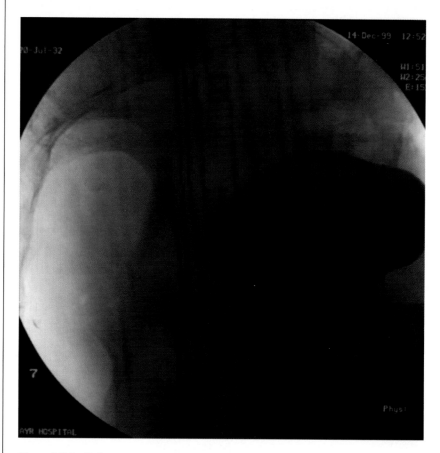

Figure 2.2.4   Follow-up cystogram

Comment

In a well motivated patient who is not septic, the use of conservative treatment for a urethro-rectal fistula, (providing there is a long fistula tract), may be successful in closing the tract and avoiding potentially hazardous open surgery and the use of a defunctioning colostomy.

Case 3: Metastatic disease or not?

A 67-year-old retired civil engineer complained of recurrent urinary tract infections. He also complained of difficulty voiding and diurnal frequency. Rectally, the prostate gland felt quite hard and irregular. The PSA was 3.3. Transrectal ultrasound and mapped biopsies were carried out. A small focus of adenocarcinoma was detected in the left peripheral zone biopsies only. The tissue was too small to formally assess but was high grade.

How would you manage this patient?

A MRI scan was performed which showed a patchy decreased signal within the posterior aspect of the outer zone of the prostate and this could represent the primary tumour. The prostate gland did not appear enlarged and the prostate capsule was well defined. Chest X-ray showed slight expansion and irregular demineralisation of the posterior aspect of the 10th rib. A bone scan was performed which showed an increased uptake in relation to the 10th rib, posteriorly on the right hand side (**Figure 2.3.1 & 2.3.2**).

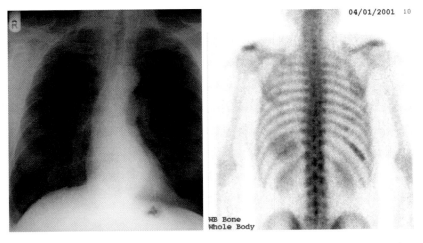

Figure 2.3.1 Chest X-ray

Figure 2.3.2 Bone scan (posterior view)

What further managment would you propose?

He appeared to have a small, localised carcinoma of the prostate, which was supported by a low PSA level. However, radiological investigation revealed an abnormality in the ribs, which could represent a metastatic deposit. Certainly, local therapy would be difficult to institute in view of this known abnormality (there had not been any previous history of trauma). It was therefore decided to refer him for partial excision of the right 10th rib and this was carried out. At surgery, there was no evidence of rib fracture and pathology did not reveal any evidence of malignancy but tissue consistent with a xanthoma/fibrous histiocytoma. Whilst these further investigations and management were being carried out, he was commenced on hormonal treatment with Casodex.

The patient is keen to proceed with local treatment. What do you recommend?

Several options would be feasible. He had small volume prostate cancer with only two out of six prostatic chippings showing less than 5% involvement by tumour and a low presenting PSA level. The probability of disease outside the capsule was therefore low. Nevertheless, on the small amount of tissue obtained, he had poorly differentiated disease. He could have been treated by a radical prostatectomy or by a radical course of external beam radiotherapy. However, he was very keen to be treated with brachytherapy, although the small focus of invasive disease was high grade. A transrectal ultrasound volume study confirmed that the tumour was confined within the capsule of the prostate (with a volume of 28 ml) and investigations confirmed the suitability for brachytherapy, which includes PSA testing. He therefore received a radioactive iodine seed implant. Postoperatively, he developed a slight urethritis and dysuria, which settled within two weeks.

He is on regular follow up which includes PSA testing (which has fallen to 0.5). It may take a year or more for the PSA to reach its lowest level. The Casodex has been discontinued.

Case 4: Bone scan for low risk disease?

A 58-year-old man presented with a one-year history of hesitancy, dribbling, poor stream and occasional dysuria. He had no haematuria. Rectal examination revealed an extremely hard and smooth prostate gland on the right side, which was very suspicious of malignancy. His PSA was within the normal range at 2.7.

How would you manage this patient?

An urgent transrectal ultrasound biopsy was carried out. Biopsies were taken from the right and left peripheral and transitional zones. The lesion on the right side felt very hard and actually bent the biopsy needle. Pathology revealed adenocarcinoma of the prostate with a double Gleason Score of 3. A MRI scan of the pelvis showed appearances in the prostate consistent with malignancy (**Figure 2.4.1**). There was no para-aortic or iliac lymphadenopathy. However, there was a 1.5 cm rounded abnormal focus within the left femoral neck and a further similar focus in the left acetabulum.

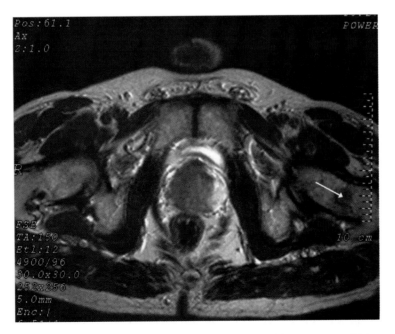

Figure 2.4.1. There is irregular bulging of the left side of the prostate, which touches the levator muscle. The prostate abuts the rectum. There is also a lesion in the neck of the left femur (arrowed)

Discuss his further management

This patient was unlikely to have bone metastases in view of the low Gleason Score and normal PSA level. In this situation, when a diagnosis of prostate cancer is made, a bone scan is not routinely performed. However, with the abnormality shown on the MRI scan, a bone scan was performed (**Figure 2.4.2 a & b**).

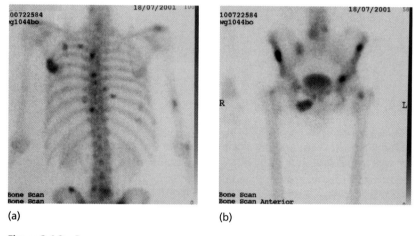

(a)   (b)

Figure 2.4.2   Bone scan

Discuss the findings and management

The bone scan showed multiple foci of increased isotope uptake throughout the axial skeleton in keeping with metastatic disease. As previously mentioned, this was surprising in view of a normal PSA level. In addition, the Gleason Score is low. He is asymptomatic from the bone metastasis but this is not unusual. He was commenced on hormonal therapy with a LHRH analogue (Zoladex) covered with a one-month course of Cyproterone acetate to protect against tumour flare. Obviously, in this situation, PSA levels cannot monitor the response to treatment. Plain X-rays of the pelvis and the right humerus were carried out which confirmed sclerotic metastases in keeping with prostate cancer. It is possible that he had bone metastases from another primary; he was a heavy smoker. However, chest X-ray was normal and the sclerotic metastases were in keeping with prostate cancer as the most likely diagnosis.

After a few months of hormonal therapy, he had fewer problems with frequency and nocturia, inferring hormone-sensitive disease. Assuming he remains asymptomatic from the bone metastases, a further bone scan should be performed in 3–6 months, which should confirm response by showing less activity. However, it is important in this situation not to perform the repeat bone scan too soon, otherwise the scan may show no change or even increased activity due to bone healing and may be wrongly interpreted as progression. The patient continues on hormonal therapy.

Footnote

The patient has been admitted within the last 2 months with bone pain and the PSA has risen to 39.4.

Comment

The pick up rate in patients with a PSA level under 10 is less than 1% (see recommended reading, page 151). In many centres, it is therefore only performed in these patients if they are symptomatic, have a raised alkaline phosphatase or if the Gleason score is 7 or more.

So, did this patient really have bone metastases from prostate cancer when the Gleason score was only 3 and the PSA was within the normal range? In retrospect it would appear so. During the most recent follow up, he has complained of bone pain, the radiology shows progression, (with increasing sclerotic metastases), and the PSA is now raised.

Case 5: Multiple urological tumours

A 70-year-old man presented with a two-year history of nocturia and frequency. This became more severe and so he was referred for urological investigation. His PSA level was elevated at 30 and a bone scan was unremarkable. A rectal examination revealed a clinically malignant gland. TURP was carried out and revealed poorly differentiated adenocarcinoma.

What treatment recommendations would you make?

This 70-year-old man appeared to have localised carcinoma of prostate. However, the PSA was quite raised and he was therefore commenced initially on hormonal therapy with Zoladex covered with Cyproterone acetate. Within three months, the PSA fell to 1.6 and arrangements were made to give a radical course of radiotherapy. A MRI scan showed disease confined to the prostate gland. He received 64 Gy in 32 fractions just over six weeks with a conformal megavoltage isocentric technique. Hormonal treatment was discontinued.

Three years later he was admitted due to haematuria causing severe anaemia. The PSA had risen to 34. He was recommenced on hormone therapy and bone scan showed increased uptake in several areas compatible with bone metastases. Cystoscopy at the time showed radiation change in the bladder alone. A further PSA level was within normal limits (0.8).

Two years later he had a further episode of haematuria. Cystoscopy revealed multiple papillary lesions in the bladder, which were resected. Histology revealed well-differentiated grade 1 papillary transitional cell carcinoma (**Figure 2.5.1a**). This can be compared with the pathology of the carcinoma of the prostate (**Figure 2.5.1b**). At the same time he had a lesion on the glans penis, which was biopsied, and this reported poorly differentiated carcinoma with focal mucin production. Immunohistochemical staining was positive for PSA and prostatic acid phosphatase (**Figure 2.5.1c**).

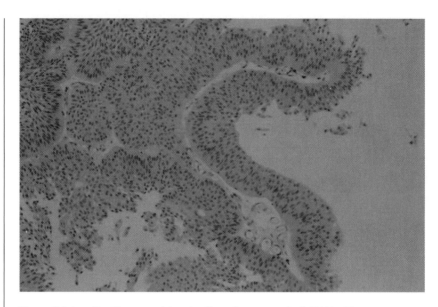

Figure 2.5.1a   Papillary transitional cell carcinoma grade 2, H&E × 32

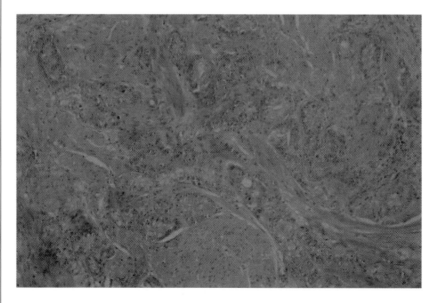

Figure 2.5.1b   Infiltrating prostatic adenocarcinoma grade 3, H&E × 32

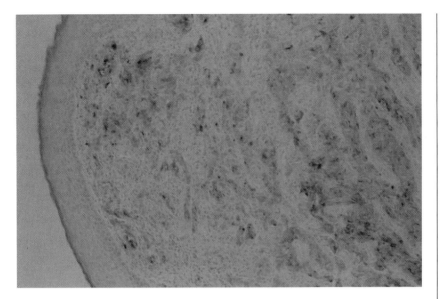

Figure 2.5.1c Glans penis biopsy with metastatic prostatic carcinoma staining positive with prostatic acid phosphatase, × 32

How would you manage this patient?

He had a good response to local therapy and hormonal treatment for carcinoma of the prostate. However, five years later he developed a new superficial bladder carcinoma as well as a deposit on the penis from prostate carcinoma. He was also known to have bone metastases at this time. The lesion on the penis had been completely resected so there was no need to give local radiotherapy to this area. He was commenced on total androgen blockade, with Casodex being added to the LHRH analogue. He had documented response to hormonal therapy at the original presentation and also three years later, and so he is likely to respond to further hormonal manipulation. However, this is likely to be for a shorter duration.

Case 6: Solitary bone metastasis

A 55-year-old road construction worker presented with urinary symptoms and a mass in the right groin. Clinical examination revealed bulky lymphadenopathy in the para-aortic region and in the right groin. He had lymphoedema of the right leg. The PSA level was elevated at 640 and histology from a transrectal biopsy revealed poorly differentiated adenocarcinoma.

How would you manage this patient?

CT scan confirmed the lymphadenopathy. He was commenced on hormonal treatment with Zoladex covered with Cyproterone acetate and the PSA level fell from 640 to 0.5. There was excellent regression of the lymphadenopathy and a reduction in the paraesthesia in his right leg and swelling. Bone scans did not show any evidence of metastatic disease.

He continued to work manually in road construction. He complained a year later of back pain, but again, a bone scan was unremarkable. After over 18 months of hormonal therapy and with a normal PSA level, the CT scan was repeated (*see* **Figure 2.6.1 a & b** comparing the serial CT scans).

Comment on the response to treatment

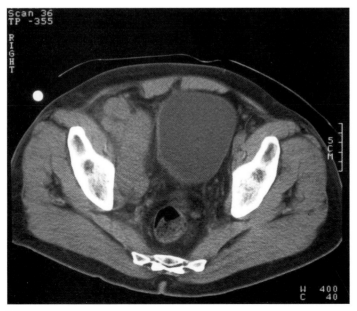

(a)

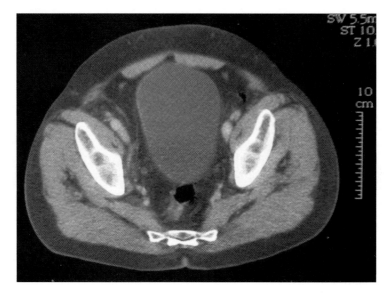

(b)

Figure 2.6.1a & b Serial CT scans

The subsequent CT scan (**Figure 2.6.1b**) shows complete resolution of the lymphadenopathy and this was supported by clinical examination. The lymphoedema of the leg had completely settled.

Would you consider a course of radiation to the pelvis at this stage?

An oncological opinion was sought, particularly regarding radiotherapy, because of an excellent response to hormonal treatment. However, it would not be possible to irradiate all the sites of previous disease and it was therefore decided to keep the patient on hormonal treatment. A year later, the PSA level started to rise slowly and he was converted to total androgen blockade.

A further year later, (over four years after his initial presentation), he complained of pain in his right shoulder. Plain X-rays of the shoulder (**Figure 2.6.2**) were taken and a bone scan was performed, (**Figure 2.6.3 a & b**). The PSA had risen to 30.

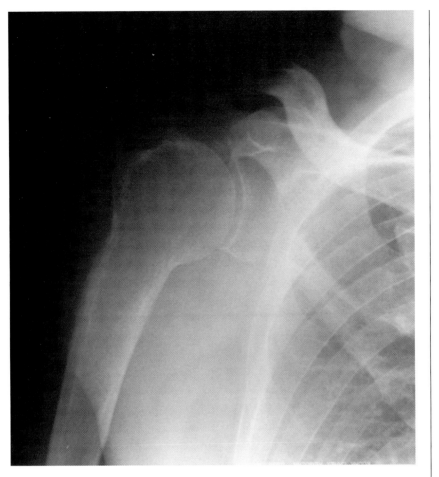

Figure 2.6.2 X-ray, right shoulder

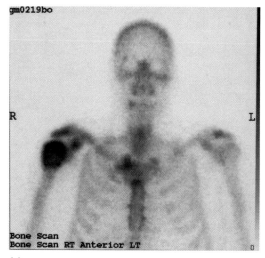

(a)

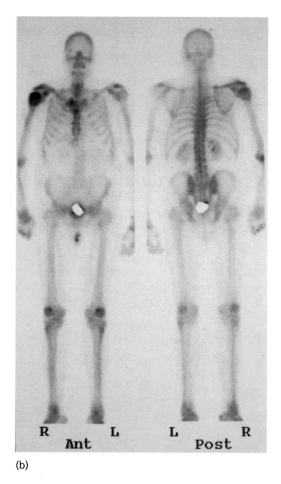

(b)

Figure 2.6.3a & b Bone scans

What management would you recommend?

Plain radiology showed a moth-eaten area in the neck of the humerus compatible with a lytic secondary, and an isotope bone scan showed a single hot spot involving the right humerus. He was referred for a specialist orthopaedic opinion but prior to attending, sustained a fracture through the surgical neck of the right humerus (**Figure 2.6.4**). He was out walking his small dog, which jerked on the lead and this caused immediate pain in his arm. X-rays showed a minimally displaced fracture through the surgical neck of the humerus. There was no evidence of neurological or vascular impairment in the right upper limb. His arm was supported in a collar and cuff and tubigrip body bandage. A trucut needle biopsy confirmed metastatic prostatic carcinoma with PSA and PAP markers positive. Subsequent X-rays showed the fracture was healing.

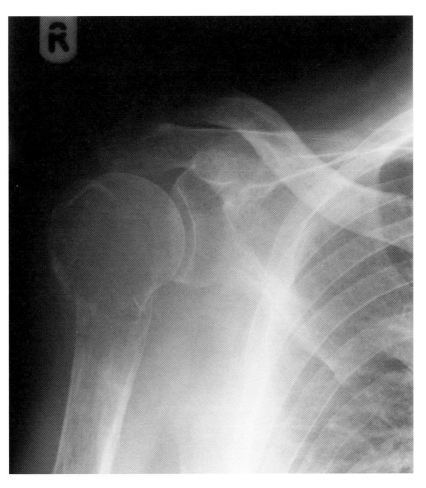

Figure 2.6.4   Subsequent shoulder X-ray

He received a course of radiotherapy to the humerus and continued on hormonal therapy. Two months later he was gradually mobilizing the right shoulder (**Figure 2.6.5**) and his pain was well controlled. The PSA level had fallen from 30 to 22.

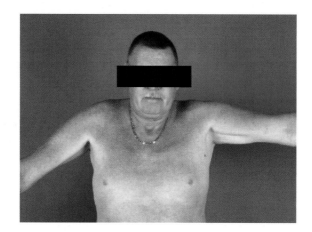

Figure 2.6.5

Comment

This case is of interest in that the patient developed a solitary bone metastasis in the humerus. It is unusual for prostate cancer to metastasise as a solitary bone metastasis, and the humerus is a most unusual site. For both of these reasons, histological confirmation was obtained prior to further management. It is also very unusual to develop a solitary bone metastasis four years after being diagnosed with metastatic prostate cancer.

Case 7: Spinal cord compression

A 64-year-old man was admitted with difficulty in walking. He had a long history of low back pain but this had become more severe, particularly over the last few months. Plain X-rays showed partial collapse of T12, mild degenerative changes and slight narrowing of the L4/5 and lumbosacral disc spaces (**Figure 2.7.1**).

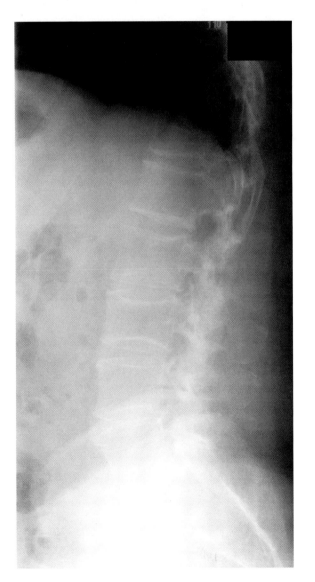

Figure 2.7.1   X-ray of lumbar spine

Clinical examination revealed a sensory level at T11/12 and reduced power in the lower limbs to 3/5. Bladder and bowel function were preserved. An urgent MRI scan and subsequent bone scan were performed.

What do these investigations show?

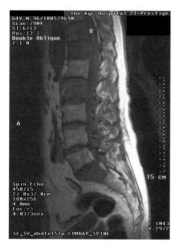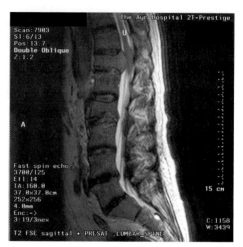

Figure 2.7.2 MRI scans

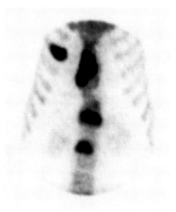

Figure 2.7.3 Bone scan

How would you manage this patient further?

The MRI scan shows partial collapse of T12 with metastatic involvement extending into the pedicles of the vertebra. There is evidence of cord compression at this level. Bone scan shows multiple hot spots in keeping with metastatic disease. The PSA level was elevated at 707.

He received a course of urgent radiotherapy to the lower thoracic spine receiving 20 Gy in five fractions over seven days. He was given high dose Dexamethasone and this was gradually tailed off. He was gradually mobilised with the aid of physiotherapy and commenced on hormonal treatment with Zoladex covered with Cyproterone acetate for the initial month.

The patient made a complete recovery from the spinal cord compression and his pain completely resolved. The PSA level fell rapidly to 0.4.

How long would you recommend LHRH therapy? Would you repeat the bone scan and if so when?

The patient remains extremely well on long term follow up. He is very reluctant to discontinue the 3 monthly injections with Zoladex. The PSA remains unrecordable at <0.2 (**Figure 2.7.4**).

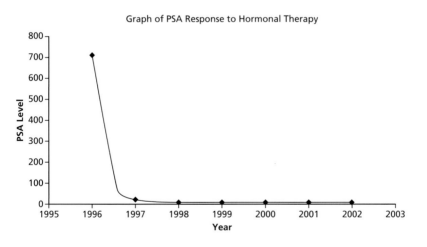

Figure 2.7.4

It may be reasonable to discontinue hormone therapy after two years and monitor the PSA level. However, whilst remaining extremely well, it was understandable that the patient wished to continue on this treatment. A further bone scan was performed three years later when he was asymptomatic in order to document response. Gratifyingly, it showed an excellent response to hormonal therapy (**Figure 2.7.5**). He remains well and symptom free six years after his original presentation.

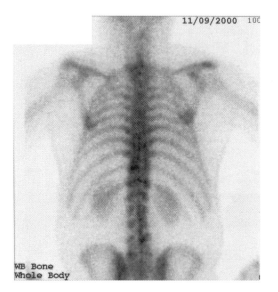

Figure 2.7.5

Comment

It is interesting that there has never been a tissue diagnosis in this patient. The prostate gland was biopsied, but no evidence of local prostate cancer found. However, he has had an amazing response to hormonal therapy and radiotherapy for widespread prostate cancer, presenting with a serious situation and a less-than-good prognosis. It is important to give prompt treatment for spinal cord pathology as some patients do surprisingly well and avoid long term neurological damage.

Case 8: Unusual sites of metastatic disease

A 45-year-old toolmaker presented with a six-month history of increasing frequency of micturition, eventually occurring up to 15 times a day. He had no haematuria. Apart from slight weight loss, he had no other complaints. He had a past medical history of epilepsy and irritable bowel disease and smoked 20 cigarettes a day. Rectal examination revealed a hard, fixed, irregular prostate gland and biopsies confirmed malignancy. His PSA level was elevated at 334.

What further investigations would you recommend and what treatment would you propose?

This relatively young man (especially with respect to carcinoma of the prostate) neglected his symptoms for several months until he had most severe frequency of micturition due to locally advanced carcinoma of the prostate. This was confirmed with a markedly elevated PSA level and biopsies of the prostate. Baseline investigations, including renal function, should be performed. Ultrasonography revealed moderate hydronephrosis of the right kidney. CT scan of the abdomen and pelvis was arranged (**Figure 2.8.1**) and bone scan revealed two areas of increased uptake in the sternum and left scapula which could have been due to metastatic disease.

What abnormalities are shown on the CT scan of the pelvis?

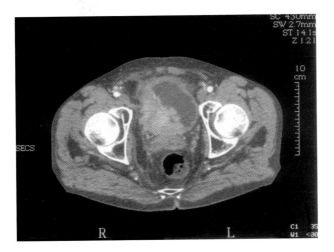

Figure 2.8.1 Pelvic CT scan

Renal function was normal. The CT scan revealed extensive pelvic tumour extending from the prostate and involving the bladder. There was evidence of both local spread into perivesical tissues and distant lymph node metastasis. He therefore had a T4 tumour. The right kidney was obstructed. This was confirmed at cystoscopy with the bladder invaded and fixed by tumour. The right ureteric orifice was also invaded by tumour and could not be cannulated. He was commenced on hormonal treatment, initially with monthly Zoladex injections covered by a course of Cyproterone acetate.

His symptoms improved markedly and the PSA level fell from 334 to 81 within two months. It continued to fall over the following few months to 10.5 but he developed left lateral chest pain and was quite tender on palpation over his ribs.

What further management would you recommend?

He was known to have widespread metastatic prostate cancer and his pain was not controlled with analgesic medication. It would have been very appropriate to give radiotherapy, as this is effective for local pain. He was given a single fraction of 8 Gy using orthovoltage (250 KV) X-rays. A further bone scan was performed, which showed various other areas of increased uptake compatible with more widespread bone metastases. As full blood count and renal function showed adequate bone marrow and renal function, he received an injection of radioactive strontium, of 150 Megabecquerels. Symptomatic improvement from bony pain may be delayed up to 8–12 weeks after radioactive strontium and thus it is often used in conjunction with local radiotherapy, as in this case. Strontium has been shown to reduce the need for subsequent local radiotherapy at other sites. Just over six months later he complained of increasing urinary symptoms, back pain and consecutive increases in the PSA level. He was commenced on Flutamide, in addition to continuing Zoladex, to achieve total androgen blockade. Casodex could also have been used as an alternative to Flutamide.

The patient tolerated this treatment well but then complained of decreased vision in his right eye over three weeks. Visual acuity in the right eye was reduced to counting fingers and a CT scan of the orbits was arranged.

What abnormalities are shown from the clinical photograph and scan (Figure 2.8.2) and what treatment would you recommend?

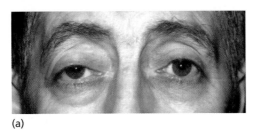

(a)

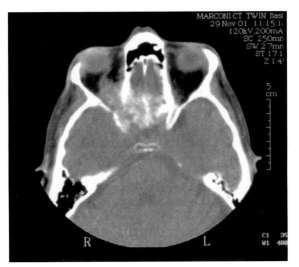

(b)

Figure 2.8.2

The clinical photograph demonstrates ptosis of the right eye. The globe was proptosed approximately 5 mm and displaced inferiorly. Movements of the right eye were restricted. The right optic disc was markedly swollen.

The CT scan shows a destructive lesion of the right orbit, with a soft tissue mass around the greater wing of the right sphenoid, extending into the right orbital apex and compressing the optic nerve. He was commenced on high-dose steroids to try and reduce the swelling and compression of the optic nerve and given an urgent course of radio-therapy. Due to the extensive nature of the deposit, he was treated with parallel-opposed radiation fields receiving 20 Gy in five fractions. The dose of steroids was rapidly tailed off and one month later there was a marked improvement in his vision and reduction in the ptosis (**Figure 2.8.3**).

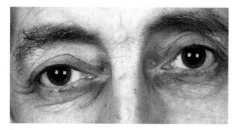

Figure 2.8.3

The patient continues on management for widespread metastatic carcinoma and his prognosis is poor.

Case 9: Prostatic cancer and liver metastases?

A 60-year-old company director presented complaining of impotence. Rectal examination revealed a hard, nodular prostate gland and a PSA level of 16. Three years earlier, he had been treated for mild bladder outflow obstruction. He had a very poor urinary flow with a high residual volume. Subsequently, a TURP was performed and histology confirmed carcinoma of the prostate (Gleason Score 8). Bone scans showed degenerative disease only.

How would you manage this patient?

Initially this gentleman was referred with mild bladder outflow obstruction symptoms and thought to have benign disease. On follow up his symptoms deteriorated. His PSA rose to a level of 16 and on a rectal examination his prostate felt quite hard and nodular. Initially it was thought that his raised PSA was related to chronic urinary sepsis. A TURP was performed, rather than a transrectal ultrasound guided biopsy, because the patient had poor flows and high residuals. This confirmed the diagnosis of a Gleason 8 prostatic carcinoma. Subsequent bone scan showed degenerative disease only.

He appeared to have a locally extensive carcinoma of the prostate but without a very markedly raised PSA level. He was commenced on hormonal treatment with a LHRH analogue covered by Cyproterone acetate. At the same time, a MRI scan of the pelvis was carried out, (**Figure 2.9.1a & b**). It revealed a large prostatic mass with changes suspicious of local invasion superiorly into the bladder and posteriorly into the pre-rectal tissues. The fat planes were lost between the rectum, seminal vesicles and prostate. There was no lymphadenopathy. Following a three-month course of hormonal therapy and clinical regression of the prostatic tumour, he was planned for a course of high-dose radiotherapy to the prostate. This was planned conformally with the aid of a CT planning scan. He received 64 Gy in 32 fractions over 45 days.

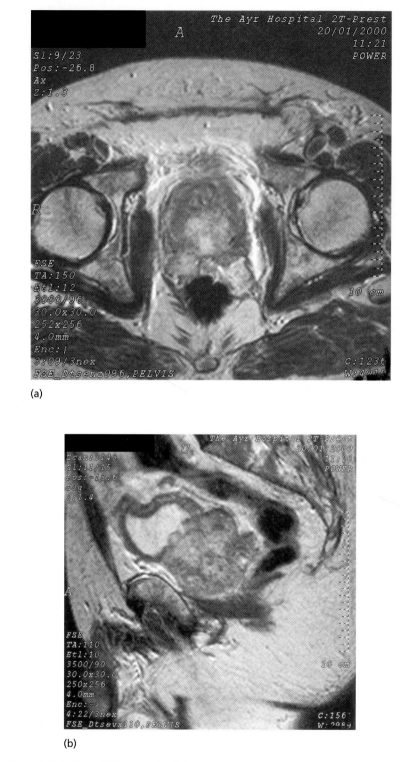

(a)

(b)

Figure 2.9.1a & b MRI scans of pelvis

Three months after completion of radiotherapy, and whilst he was still on LHRH analogue injections, the PSA level was 5.8. However, a month later, he continued to have vague complaints and abdominal discomfort. He was very anxious. Clinical examination was satisfactory. Liver function tests were slightly abnormal and liver ultrasound revealed lesions in the liver compatible with metastatic disease (**Figure 2.9.2**).

What management would you recommend?

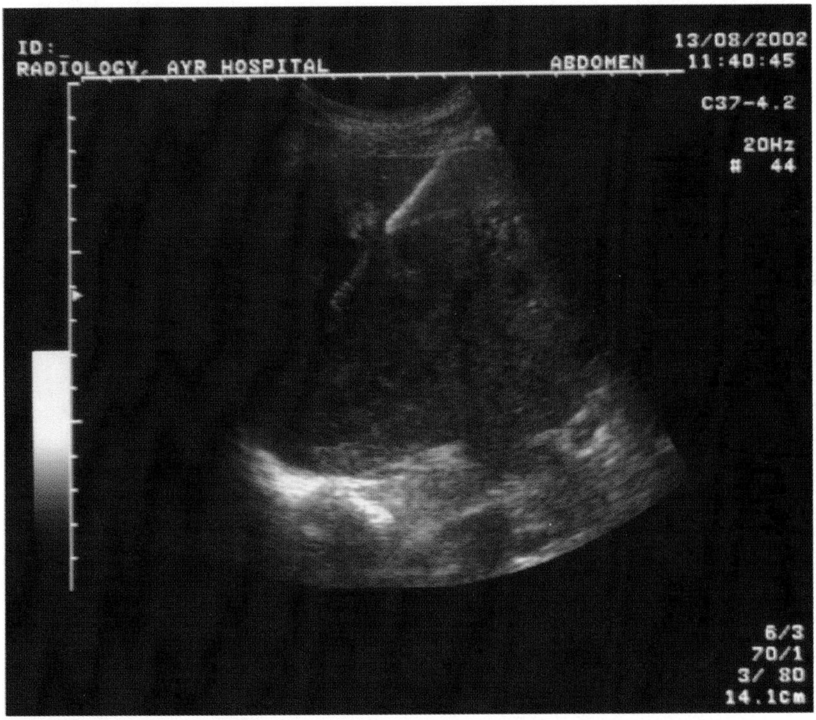

Figure 2.9.2

Liver biopsy was performed under ultrasound control and following checking of normal clotting factors. Pathology of both the prostate (**Figure 2.9.3**) and liver (**Figure 2.9.4**) are shown below.

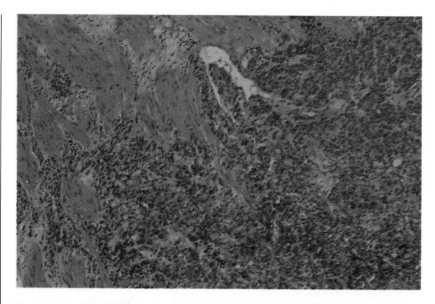

Figure 2.9.3   Prostatic carcinoma infiltrating muscle in the prostate, H&E × 32

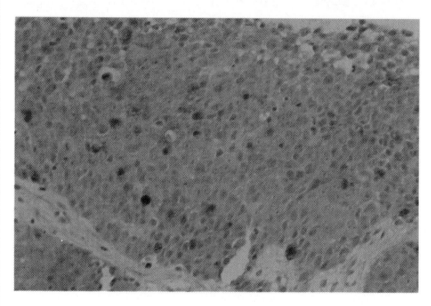

Figure 2.9.4   Metastatic carcinoma in the liver, weakly positive staining for prostatic specific antigen, × 64

What is your interpretation and recommendations?

It would be very unusual for prostate cancer to metastasise to the liver. It was therefore important to confirm the diagnosis with a liver biopsy. The biopsy needle *in situ* can be seen on the ultrasound scan. The biopsy showed large pleomorphic cells having large vesicular nuclei. No mucin could be demonstrated. Prostatic markers showed occasional positive cells but not the typical pattern one would expect with prostate cancer. The appearances were essentially of an undifferentiated large cell carcinoma and pathologically, the lung might be a possible primary site. It was felt to be unlikely to have arisen from the gastrointestinal tract in the absence of mucin.

Both clinically and on further investigation, there was no evidence of a lung primary. He was a non-smoker. The patient was very keen to have active management with chemotherapy. Chemotherapy for prostate cancer is not widely used and it is not very chemosensitive, so it did not seem sensible to treat him with a chemotherapy regime such as Mitoxantrone and Prednisolone, or a taxoid. He sought a second opinion and received chemotherapy using a combination chemotherapy regimen to cover a lung primary. It was very unlikely that he would have a good response and indeed he died three months later.

Case 10: Bone marrow infiltration

A 67-year-old retired medical colleague presented complaining of mild frequency of micturition, nocturia and reduced urinary flow. Rectal examination revealed a small, hard nodular prostate gland and the PSA level was raised at 169.6. TRUS biopsies of both sides of the gland were carried out and revealed poorly differentiated adenocarcinoma with a Gleason Score of 10. Bone scan was normal. CT scan showed appearances compatible with a tumour in the prostate gland and a large pelvic lymph node (**Figure 2.10.1**).

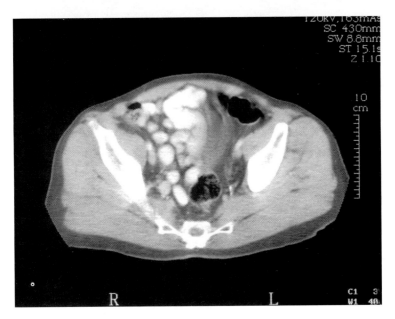

Figure 2.10.1   CT scan of pelvis

What management would you recommend?

The patient has high-risk disease with a markedly elevated PSA level and a high Gleason Score. It is likely that the imaging is indicative of a pelvic node involvement. A MR lymphangiogram was performed using Sinerem (iron oxide nanoparticles in low molecular dextran). These are taken up by macrophages, particularly within lymph nodes. Metastatic nodes, where macrophages have been replaced by tumour, do not take up iron, hence there is no signal drop. This showed an enlarged pelvic lymph node (**Figure 2.10.2**) with no contrast uptake, (which in over 85% of cases is diagnostic of nodal involvement). He was commenced on Zoladex with Cyproterone acetate cover and the PSA level fell rapidly to 1.5. He wished to proceed with a course of high-dose radiotherapy to the prostate gland, in spite of the fact that he was at very high risk of having metastatic disease. He received 64 Gy in 32 fractions using conformal radiotherapy with a 4 field megavoltage isocentric technique.

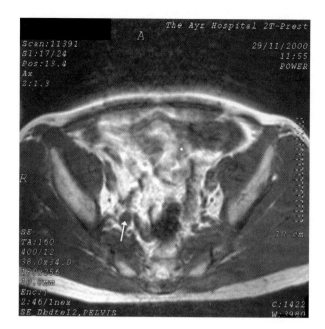

Figure 2.10.2 MRI scan of pelvis

Three months after completing radiotherapy the PSA had risen to 94.9. He was asymptomatic apart from low back pain for which he took simple analgesic medication.

What further management would you recommend?

He was commenced on total androgen blockade by adding Casodex and a bone scan arranged (**Figure 2.10.3 a–c**). He was considered for radioactive Strontium but a full blood count showed a marked thrombocytopenia.

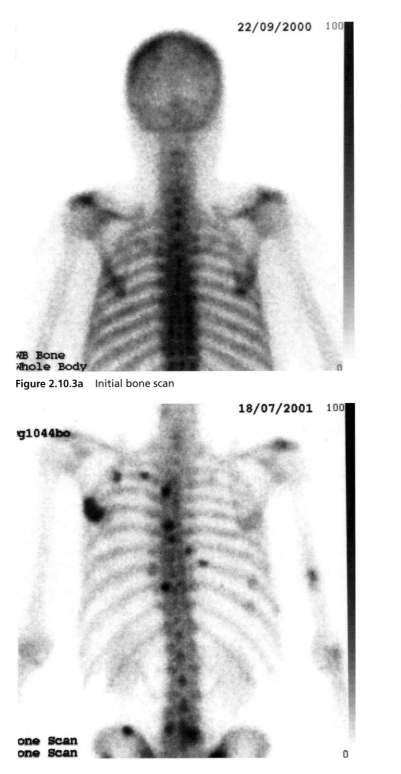

22/09/2000

WB Bone
Whole Body

Figure 2.10.3a Initial bone scan

18/07/2001

g1044bo

one Scan
one Scan

Figure 2.10.3b Follow up bone scan

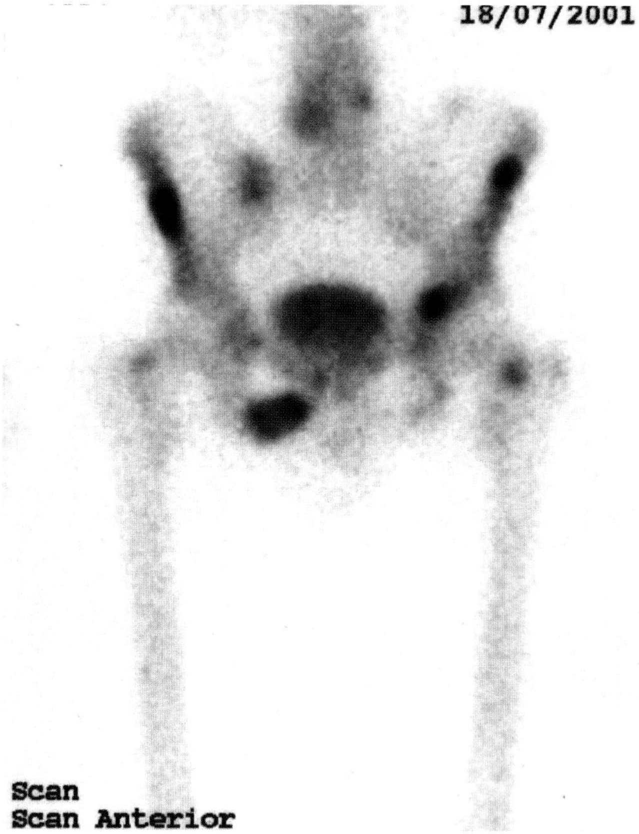

18/07/2001

Scan
Scan Anterior

Figure 2.10.3c Follow up bone scan

What further management would you recommend?

He had a full coagulation screen, which showed a low fibrinogen and the platelet count was checked and confirmed to be low. He was instructed to stop Ibuprofen, which may exacerbate thrombocytopenia and advised to take Paracetamol. He was commenced on Dexamethasone, which stabilised the thrombocytopenia and he did not require regular blood transfusions. However, several months later, he did require more platelet support and cryoprecipitate to try and reduce the extent of bruising and bleeding due to disseminated intravascular coagulation. Low dose Fragmin was also employed to try and reduce the DIC.

He had been supported haematologically for six months from detection of his thrombocytopenia, when he became breathless on minimal exertion and further investigation revealed this was due to multiple pulmonary emboli, which was a terminal event.

SECTION 3: KIDNEY

Case 1   Adapting treatment for an unusual situation   73
Case 2   Management of a complex renal cyst   77
Case 3   The equivocal renal tumour   81
Case 4   Surveillance of the upper urinary tract   85
Case 5   Immunotherapy sensitive renal carcinoma   91
Case 6   The role of surgery   97
Case 7   Metastatic disease; unknown primary   101

Case 1: Adapting treatment for an unusual situation

A 45-year-old lady was referred by her GP for an outpatient ultra-sound because of abdominal pain. When she attended, she was in severe pain and ultrasound showed a large right-sided renal mass. This was interpreted as an angiomyelolipoma of the kidney with areas of thrombus. There appeared to be a large aneurysm at the lower pole associated with evidence of fresh bleeding. The lady was admitted as an emergency. She had an obvious palpable and pulsatile abdominal mass.

How would you proceed with the management of this patient?

What does the CT scan (Figure 3.1.1) demonstrate?

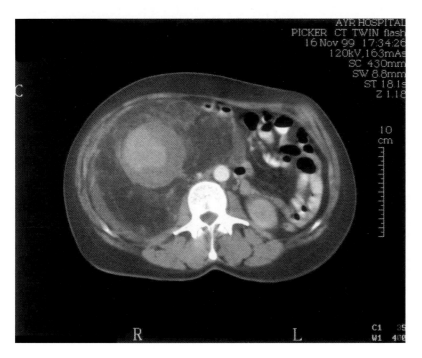

Figure 3.1.1 Abdominal CT scan

A CT scan was performed and showed greatly increased perirenal fat that extended across the midline, displacing bowel to the left. The 7 cm lesion within the fat was an aneurysm arising from the lower pole of the right kidney. Stranding within the perinephric fat and thickening of the perinephric fascia posteriorly was in keeping with recent haemorrhage. It confirmed and clarified the ultrasound findings.

The patient was haemodynamically stable but her CT scans had confirmed the fact that she was bleeding at the site of the aneursymal blood vessel into the angiomyelolipoma. Angiography was arranged and the main feeding vessel to the angiomyelolipoma was identified and embolised. Later, at laparotomy, the main blood supply to the angiomyelolipoma was found to be arising just above the bifurcation of the aorta. The large venous plexus connecting directly to the inferior vena cava and emanating from the tumour mass was individually ligated. The mass itself was adherent to the posterior part of the kidney. It was not possible to dissect this from the kidney and so nephrectomy and removal of the large mass were performed (**Figure 3.1.2**). The patient made an uneventful postoperative recovery.

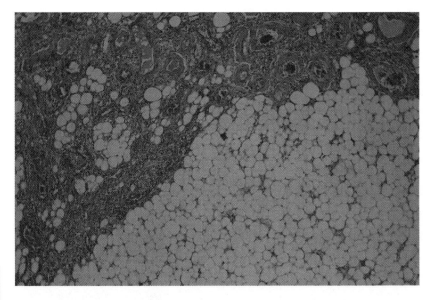

Figure 3.1.2 Angiomyclolipoma showing mixture of blood vessels, cellular stroma and fat cells H&E × 12.8

What further investigations would you organise?

A CT scan of brain was performed to make sure that she did not have any associated cerebral abnormalities. This was normal. Apparently, the patient had been complaining of migraines and headaches before admission.

Comment

The emergency procedure was done in collaboration with a vascular surgeon. The delineation of the blood supply to the angiomyelolipoma was extremely helpful and embolisation prior to surgery made the dissection less hazardous. The patient requires long-term surveillance of the other kidney to ensure she does not develop any other angio-myelolipomatous lesions. Four years following her surgery she remains well.

Case 2: Management of a complex renal cyst

A well, fit 50-year-old lady had vague abdominal pain investigated. Her GP organised an abdominal ultrasound. She had no urinary symptoms and no haematuria. The ultrasound showed a 6 × 6 cm cystic mass with multiple septi arising from the equatorial part of the right kidney. The appearance of the complex renal cyst was thought to represent a simple haemorrhagic cyst, although more sinister pathology could not be excluded.

How would you manage the patient?

The patient was referred for a CT scan (**Figure 3.2.1**). The mass was confirmed as a cystic lesion, which had multiple loculations and no marked wall thickening. There were no other abnormalities and particularly no lymphadenopathy. The lesion was again thought to be a complex cyst but it was not entirely possible on radiological grounds to exclude a tumour.

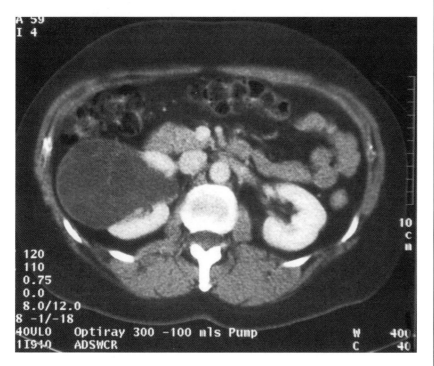

Figure 3.2.1   CT scan of abdomen

What further management would you propose?

She was a fit middle-aged woman. Should biopsy or aspiration of the cyst have been performed? A negative cytology report would not definitely exclude a renal tumour. The other kidney was entirely normal and so, following lengthy discussion with the patient, she proceeded to nephrectomy. An alternative approach would have been to carry out serial ultrasound and CT scans to see if there was any change in the large cystic lesion.

The possibility of partial nephrectomy was excluded by the fact that the complex cyst extended across the equatorial region of the kidney and into the renal pelvis, making it technically not feasible. The patient had a standard radical nephrectomy through a supracostal incision and made a gradual recovery.

This lady had a very unusual tumour. She had a multiloculated cystic nephroma (**Figure 3.2.2**). This is a rare and benign renal tumour. The appearances on the pathological specimen complement those of the radiological investigations.

Was this the correct management of the patient?

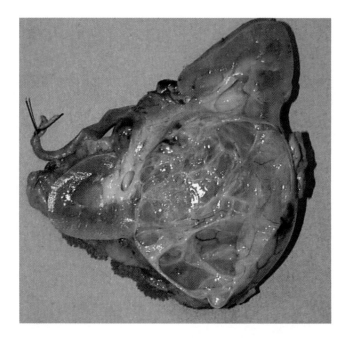

Figure 3.2.2   Transected kidney with multilobulated cystic tumour

Performing a radical procedure for a patient who ends up having a benign lesion is always a concern regarding the potential morbidity and threat to life of the surgery. However, this has to be balanced by the fact that, with these types of lesions, there is always ongoing concern by the patient, the surgeon and the radiologist as to whether adopting conservative surveillance is in the best interests of the patient. Had this lesion turned out to be a cystic renal cell cancer (as it may well have been from its appearance on imaging), then surveillance may have been to the detriment of this patient. The management of these complex cysts is difficult clinically, as it is not always possible to give the patient a definitive answer before surgery as to whether they have a renal carcinoma or just a benign cyst. Surgery should only be undertaken with the understanding of the patient concerning this medical dilemma.

Case 3: The equivocal renal tumour

A healthy active 76-year-old gentleman regularly attended his GP because of difficulty in controlling his blood pressure. He was noted to have an abdominal mass, which was confirmed, on ultrasound, to be renal in origin. A CT scan of the abdomen confirmed a very large mass (13.7 × 10 × 13.6 cm) involving the mid and lower pole of the right kidney (**Figure 3.3.1**). There was no evidence of invasion of the renal vein and no significant lymphadenopathy. The left kidney was normal, as was the chest X-ray.

How would you manage this patient?

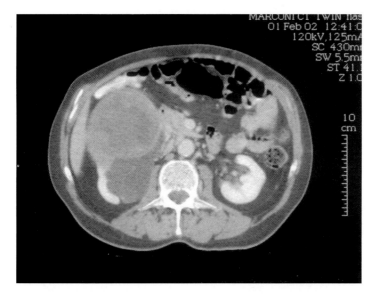

Figure 3.3.1 The CT shows a large tumour mass projecting from the anterior surface of the right kidney. The tumour is compressing the upper ureter and causing hydronephrosis

It may be appropriate in the elderly patient to treat localised renal carcinoma conservatively but clearly in an active, well man, (who regularly played golf) surgery was indicated. The patient underwent a right radical nephrectomy through a supra-costal incision. There was no obvious hilar lymphadenopathy and the adrenal gland was left as the renal lesion involved only the equatorial and lower pole area. Post-operatively, the patient made an uneventful recovery.

Pathologically, there was no evidence of tumour through the renal capsule (**Figure 3.3.2**) and no evidence of any hilar lymphadepathy. The histological pattern was not that of a typical renal cell carcinoma but of a carcinoma with acinar and ductular morphology with some areas showing more papillary architecture. The overall features were consistent with a papillary renal cell carcinoma (**Figure 3.3.3**). There was no involvement of any vascular channel and the renal vein itself was clear. The cut margin of the ureter showed no abnormality.

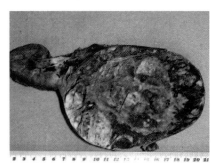

Figure 3.3.2   Large renal tumour involving the lower pole of the kidney

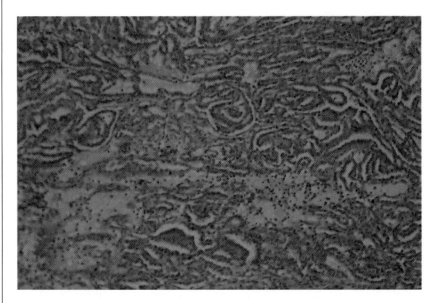

Figure 3.3.3   Papillary renal cell carcinoma showing foamy cells, H&E × 32

How should this patient be followed up?

Papillary renal cell carcinoma has a slightly better prognosis than clear cell carcinoma. This was classified as type A papillary renal cell carcinoma. However, these tumours are more frequently multi-focal and bilateral than typical clear cell renal cancers. Despite his age, he requires regular follow up with radiology of the remaining kidney on an annual basis.

Case 4: Surveillance of the upper urinary tract

A 51-year-old well lady presented with haematuria and was diagnosed as having a single papillary tumour, which was a superficial transitional cell cancer of the bladder PTa G1. She was put on regular cystoscopic surveillance following initial resection and at her first cystoscopy four months later there was no recurrence. She had small recurrences that were diathermied in the subsequent year and further small recurrences four and eight years later.

Is this adequate surveillance?

This patient remained asymptomatic. She had no episodes of haematuria apart from at presentation and the IVP showed no disease in the upper urinary tract. In some urological units, it would be standard protocol to monitor the upper tracts by regular IVPs, as there is a clear association with the development of further upper tract tumours. This is also now our policy.

Ten years later she developed further severe haematuria following a recent check cystoscopy, which showed no bladder recurrence.

How would you manage this patient?

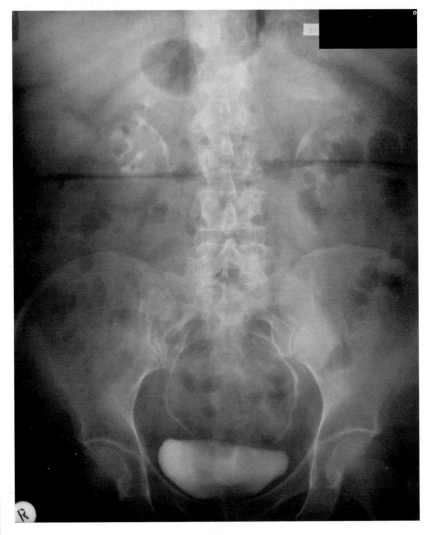

Figure 3.4.1 The IVU film shows irregularity of the inferior margin of the right renal pelvis

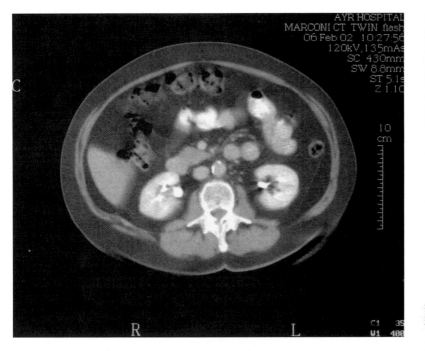

Figure 3.4.2   The CT scan confirms an irregular filling defect within the renal pelvis

Radiological investigation with an IVU (**Figure 3.4.1**) and CT scan (**Figure 3.4.2**) revealed a large filling defect in the right renal pelvis. The left kidney was entirely normal.

How would you surgically manage this patient?

The lesion in the right renal pelvis measured $2 \times 2 \times 1$ cm. It would have been possible to undertake conservative treatment with flexible urethroscopy and laser ablation of the tumour. This would almost certainly have required repeated procedures. The other option would have been a right nephroureterectomy. The former option is usually reserved for patients with compromised contralateral renal function. The patient therefore underwent a right radical nephroureterectomy and made an uneventful recovery. Pathology is shown below (**Figure 3.4.3** and **Figure 3.4.4**).

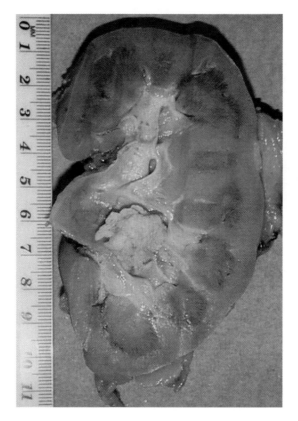

Figure 3.4.3 Sectioned kidney to show polypoid mass in the lower calyx

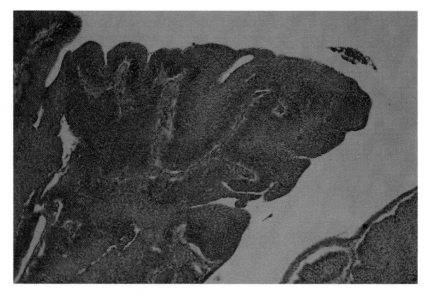

Figure 3.4.4 Papillary transitional cell carcinoma Grade 2, H&E × 12.8

Comment

In a busy urological department, cystoscopic surveillance of patients with transitional cell bladder tumours is a major part of the workload. It is all too easy to forget the upper tracts during this surveillance process and it is important that departments establish and adhere to protocols for follow up.

Case 5: Immunotherapy sensitive renal carcinoma

A 48-year-old man presented with weight loss, malaise, abdominal pain, dysuria and haematuria. Investigations, including a CT scan, were performed.

What abnormality does this show?

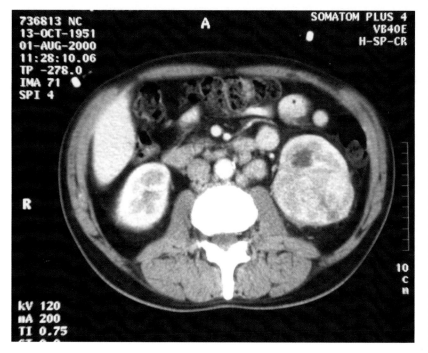

Figure 3.5.1 CT scan of abdomen

What management would you propose?

The CT scan of the abdomen showed a large left sided renal carcinoma. The tumour appeared to be confined to the kidney. There was no lymphadenopathy. Further investigations did not reveal any evidence of metastatic disease.

A left nephrectomy was performed and pathology revealed a tumour with extensive necrosis and haemorrhage. Most of the tumour consisted of pleomorphic rather than papillary clear cell carcinoma (**Figure 3.5.2**). The tumour extended beyond the renal capsule into the perinephric fat. The tumour was vascular but there was no definite invasion of blood vessels and the hilum was free of tumour. There was evidence of tumour protruding into the ureter. Lymph nodes in the vicinity of the tumour, which were excised, showed no evidence of tumour.

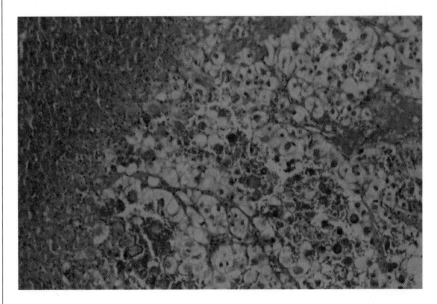

Figure 3.5.2 Renal cell carcinoma nuclear grade 4 (with necrosis on the right side), H&E × 32

Four months later, the patient was admitted due to further weight loss and anaemia and a further CT scan was performed.

What does this show (Figure 3.5.3)?

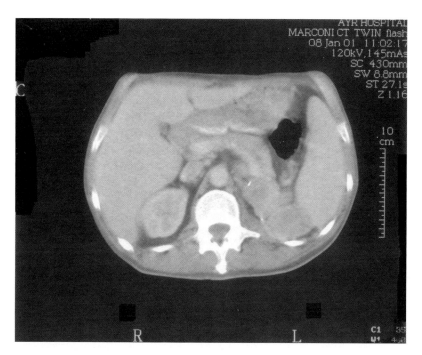

Figure 3.5.3   Follow up CT scan after surgery

How would you manage him now?

This CT scan showed an irregular soft tissue mass in the left renal bed measuring $8 \times 4 \times 4$ cm and multiple enlarged para–aortic and aortocaval lymph nodes, most measuring 1 cm.

He was commenced on treatment with Interferon, initially starting at 3 MU three times a week and escalating the dose after a week to 6 MU and then 9 MU. He tolerated this treatment well. After six months therapy, a further CT scan was arranged to document response.

What does this show (Figure 3.5.4)? How do you explain the appearances?

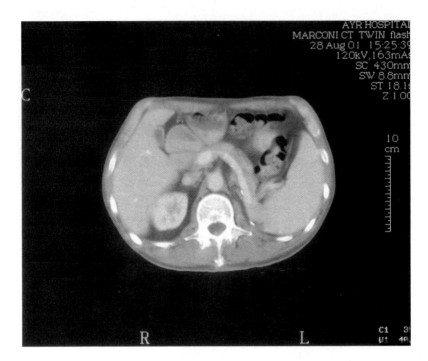

Figure 3.5.4   Further CT scan after Interferon treatment for 6 months

The patient felt very well on Interferon and felt that he was responding to therapy. He had less fatigue and was putting on weight. The CT scan showed excellent resolution of the changes, particularly in the left renal bed. It appeared that he had had a very good response to Interferon therapy. Radiology was reviewed in view of the surprisingly good response. The appearances at re-presentation could have been due to postoperative change but they are far more in keeping with tumour recurrence. In addition, the patient's symptoms improved markedly, supporting the assumption that tumour regression has ocurred.

After a further three months of Interferon therapy and at routine review, although he remained well, he was leucopenic (white cell count $2.3 \times 10^9/L$) and thrombocytopenic (platelet count $40 \times 10^9/L$).

What would you suggest?

These blood count changes could have been due to Interferon therapy and it was therefore stopped. Myelosuppression is a known side effect of Interferon. As he remained extremely well, a less likely scenario could be bone marrow infiltration by renal carcinoma. After being off Interferon for two months, the white count had recovered but the platelet count was still reduced, although improved $(76 \times 10^9/\text{L})$. A further CT scan was carried out and this showed very little change (**Figure 3.5.5**). The patient remains well and off therapy at present.

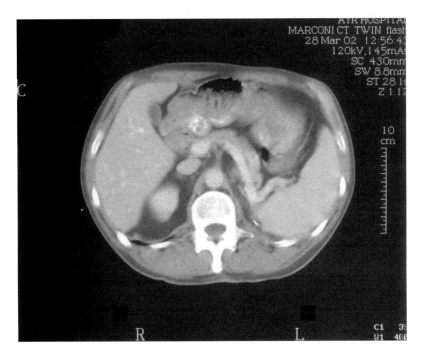

Figure 3.5.5 CT scan having discontinued Interferon

Case 6: The role of surgery

A 60-year-old, self-employed heating engineer presented with a few months history of anorexia, half-a-stone weight loss and malaise. He had two episodes of haematuria. Clinical examination was unremarkable. Investigations included IVU and CT scan (**Figure 3.6.1** and **Figure 3.6.2**).

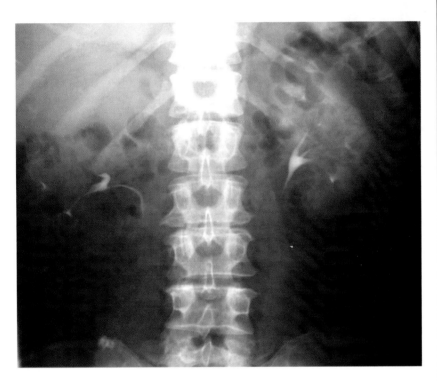

Figure 3.6.1   Intravenous urogram

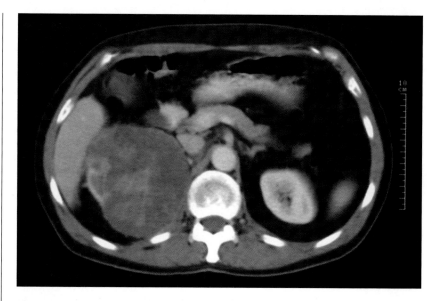

Figure 3.6.2 CT scan of abdomen

What do these investigations show? How would you manage this patient?

Baseline blood tests were normal although his ESR was raised at 90. Together with the above symptoms, this was suggestive of a malignancy. The IVU showed a large mass in the upper pole of the right kidney, distorting and displacing the mid and lower pole calyces. An ultrasound scan confirmed that this was a solid lesion. Similar appearances were shown on the CT scan. The lower pole of the right kidney was displaced inferiorly. The mass was well defined, extending posteriorly into the right posterior para-renal space and immediately applied to the right crus and right adjacent posterior abdominal wall. There was no involvement of the IVC and the right renal vein may have been involved but was not clearly identified. There was no lymphadenopathy and no evidence of spread into the chest.

The tumour was likely to be operable and he therefore underwent a right nephrectomy. Histology showed a typical renal carcinoma of clear cell pattern with penetration of the renal capsule and invasion of the right renal vein. Hilar and peri renal lymph nodes were not involved. He did not receive any further treatment at this time.

A year later, he complained of discomfort in the right costal margin and upper abdominal pain. Clinical examination was satisfactory. A chest X-ray and bone scan were normal but a CT scan showed a small circular opacity in the right lower lobe. There was no other abnormality.

How would you manage this patient?

It was likely that he had developed a solitary metastasis from renal carcinoma. He had high-risk disease in that the renal vein was invaded and there was penetration of the capsule. He had already had a reasonable disease-free period and so a right thoracotomy and wedge excision was considered. This procedure was then carried out and pathology confirmed recurrent clear cell carcinoma.

At review six months later, he remained asymptomatic but a routine follow up CT scan was performed which showed a large subcarinal mass of lymph nodes. He also had a few deposits in both lungs shown on CT scan.

How would you manage this patient now?

He was well and asymptomatic but wanted active therapy. Observation could have been an option but he wanted more active management. He was therefore commenced on Medroxyprogesterone acetate (300 mg / day). This hormonal treatment was compared with Interferon in the REO1 MRC trial and found to be inferior, but as he was asymptomatic and was treated several years ago, this management was chosen as initial therapy. Subsequent chest X-rays and one CT scan have been very satisfactory with complete regression of the pulmonary metastases and lymphadenopathy.

He remains well five years later and continues on Medroxyprogesterone acetate. This illustrates an excellent response of metastatic renal carcinoma to hormonal therapy. It also demonstrates the value of dealing with an isolated metastic deposit from renal carcinoma surgically, although he did develop mediastinal lymphadenopathy six months later.

Case 7: Metastatic disease; unknown primary

A 53-year-old development officer was admitted with a two-month history of cough productive of white sputum, shortness of breath and feeling very unwell with marked weight loss. He had no pain. On examination at presentation, he had signs consistent with a large pleural effusion. He smoked 10 cigarettes a day. Chest X-ray was carried out and is shown in figure 3.7.1.

What does this show?

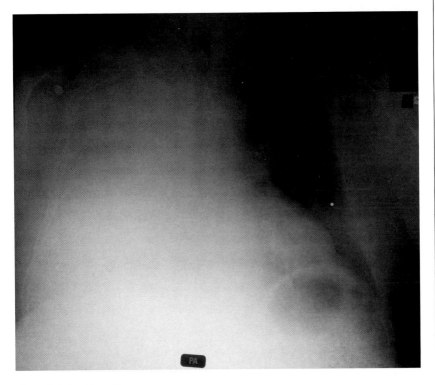

Figure 3.7.1 Chest X-ray

How would you manage this patient further?

Clinically, he had signs consistent with a large pleural effusion and this was confirmed on chest X-ray. Therefore, pleural drainage with the insertion of an intercostal drain was performed. Heavily bloodstained fluid drained freely. As is often the case with heavily bloodstained fluid, no malignant cells were identified, but the fact that it was heavily blood-stained made malignancy highly likely.

A CT scan was performed of the chest and abdomen following drainage of the pleural effusion. What does this show? (Figure 3.7.2)

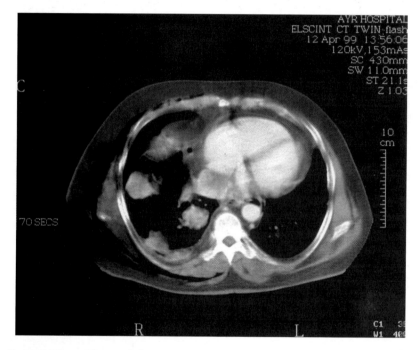

Figure 3.7.2 a   CT scan of chest

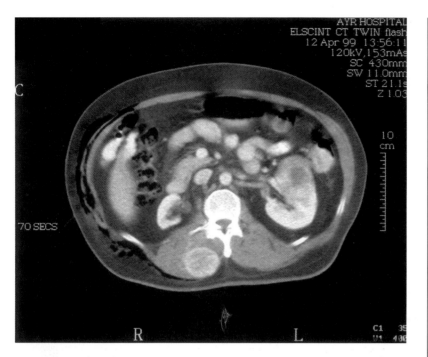

Figure 3.7.2 b   CT scan of abdomen

The scan showed multiple intrapulmonary lesions consistent with metastases and, in addition, multiple enhancing soft tissue masses of varying sizes involving the erector spinae muscles, the right gluteus majoris muscles bilaterally and subcutaneous fat in the buttock on the left side in keeping with secondary deposits. There was a mass in the left kidney. Bronchoscopy revealed a polypoid lesion in the anterior segment of the left upper lobe bronchus, which was also probably a secondary. The pleural fluid was an exudate but failed to yield malignant cells and a trucut biopsy of the soft tissue mass in the left gluteal region was carried out. This showed infiltration by metastatic clear cell carcinoma consistent with a primary in the kidney.

What further management would you recommend for this patient?

He had very widespread and aggressive metastatic carcinoma of the kidney. He was a relatively young man and was therefore commenced on Interferon therapy starting with 3 MU injections, 3 times a week and escalating up to 9 MU, 3 times a week. He tolerated this treatment well and a further review chest X-ray was taken over a year later (**Figure 3.7.3 a & b**).

Comment on the changes on the serial X-rays

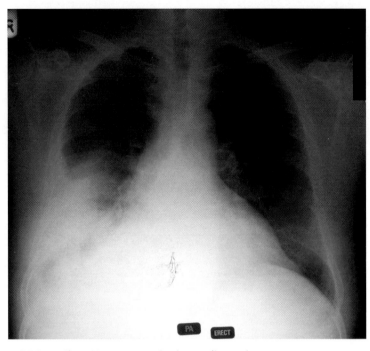

Figure 3.7.3 a Chest X-ray post aspiration at diagnosis

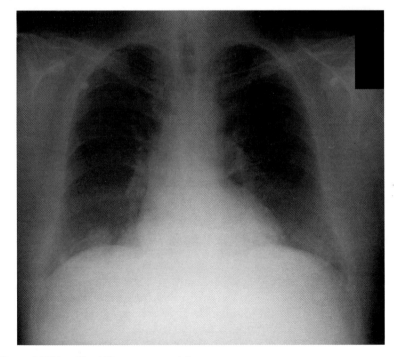

Figure 3.7.3 b Chest X-ray one year later

He had an excellent response to Interferon therapy. After the initial pleural aspiration and drainage he did not require any further pleural aspiration between these two CXR films. Despite presenting with widespread aggressive disease, as manifest by a heavily bloodstained pleural effusion, he had an excellent response to Interferon therapy, which was maintained for over a year.

SECTION 4: PENIS

Case 1   *In situ* disease   109
Case 2   The unusual location   111
Case 3   The unusual tumour   113
Case 4   Primary or metastatic?   115

Case 1: *In situ* disease

This 69-year-old man was referred with a flat erythematous lesion localised to the glans penis. It was poorly demarcated. There was slight discharge from the ulcerated area and very occasional bleeding. There was no inguinal lymphadenopathy. A biopsy was taken which revealed extensive squamous carcinoma *in situ* (**Figure 4.1.1**). Excision was not complete.

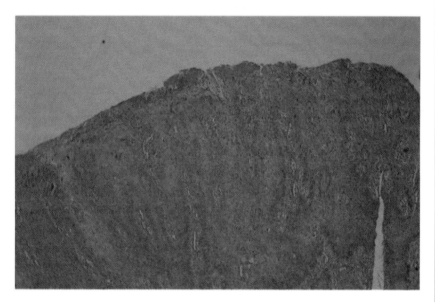

Figure 4.1.1 Thickened epidermis with carcinoma *in situ*, H&E × 12.8

How would you manage this patient?

The patient was referred for an oncological opinion, particularly with regard to radiotherapy. However, squamous carcinoma *in situ* is not radiosensitive and it is inappropriate to carry out this form of treatment. The patient was treated with Efudex cream (topical preparation of 5-Flurouracil). This has to be applied carefully by the patient using a spatula and gloves. Initially, it was applied once or twice daily for a couple of weeks. It was likely that a brisk reaction would occur. The area of disease became less active and crusted. However, due to the extensive nature of his disease, he developed a meatal stenosis requiring dilatation.

He maintained a good response to treatment with Efudex cream and the area on the penis regressed considerably. However, he later developed a more active area of disease with a more solid lesion on the left side of the glans.

How would you manage this situation?

It is important that patients are followed up carefully as they may develop frankly invasive disease. More radical treatment would then be appropriate. The area was re-excised to exclude invasive disease. Histology of the nodule again reported superficial ulcerated squamous carcinoma *in situ*. Excision was complete.

Further recurrences have occurred over the ensuing seven years and have been managed by re-excision and grafting the area with split skin graft. On every occasion, *in situ* disease has been reported with no evidence of invasive carcinoma.

Case 2: The unusual location

A 57-year-old man originally presented 3 years ago with a lesion on his penis. Apparently, topical cream was prescribed by his GP and the lesion resolved. However, it had recently progressed and he was referred for further investigation. Circumcision was performed when he was young. He had no occupational risk factors or history of note. Clinical examination revealed a lesion on the shaft of the penis measuring 4.3 × 3.5 cm and extending onto the scrotum (**Figure 4.2.1**). There was no lymphadenopathy.

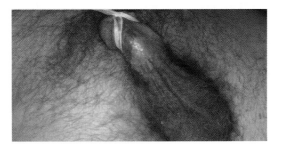

Figure 4.2.1

How would you manage and treat this patient?

Presumably, he had previously been treated by his GP for a fungal infection but it is possible, although unlikely, that the GP would have treated him with Efudex cream. Biopsy was performed and this revealed a well-differentiated infiltrating squamous carcinoma. Investigations did not reveal any evidence of metastatic disease.

Surgery would have been an option but it was not going to be possible to conserve the penis. It was therefore decided to treat the patient with a radical course of radiotherapy. Often, radiotherapy for penile lesions is carried out using a wax block and parallel-opposed fields. However, because of the location of the tumour at the base of the penis and extending onto the scrotum, this technique was not feasible. Similarly, using a radioactive implant would have been difficult and probably poorly tolerated by the scrotal tissues. A special electron cut out was therefore made and careful attention paid to the reproducibility of set up. The penis was carefully taped up so that the lesion at the base of the penis was just treated with a margin. A few millimetres of build-up was employed over the field to ensure full dose at the surface. The patient received just over 60 Gy over 30 weeks with electrons.

The patient developed a marked skin reaction with moist desquamation (**Figure 4.2.2a**), as expected, and was given instructions and careful supportive care. Two weeks after completion of radiotherapy the area was healing well. There was initial erythema and later some atrophic changes of the skin (**Figure 4.2.2b**).

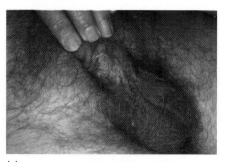

(a)

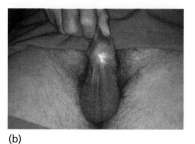

(b)

Figure 4.2.2 a & b   Follow up clinical photographs

Follow-up over 10 years revealed no evidence of recurrence. At this point the patient was discharged from the clinic. There was telangiectasia over the treated area as expected.

Case 3: The unusual tumour

A 60-year-old man presented with a large mass arising from under-neath the foreskin. He had been unable to retract the foreskin. He had noticed this swelling for several weeks but only sought medical attention when there was a discharge. It caused discomfort but no pain and he had no urinary symptoms. Clinical examination revealed a hard, irregular mass measuring 5 × 4 × 3 cm under the foreskin. There was no inguinal lymphadenopathy. Biopsies revealed an osteosarcoma. (**Figure 4.3.1**)

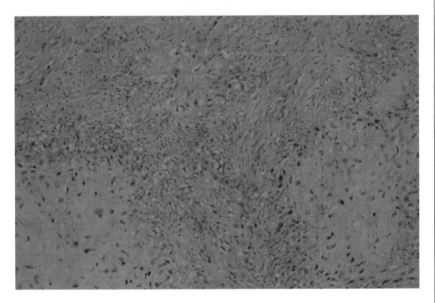

Figure 4.3.1 a Osteosarcoma of the penis with area of malignant cartilage, H&E × 32

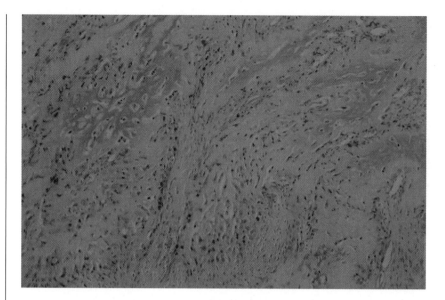

Figure 4.3.1 b   Osteosarcoma of the penis with area of osteoid formation, H&E ×
32

You are asked for an oncological opinion on the further management. What do you advise?

This was an extremely rare and unusual tumour occurring from a soft
tissue site. Histology therefore needed to be carefully reviewed. The cells
were totally negative for cytokeratin and tissue was tested for S100 to
exclude melanoma. A lot of collagen and bone were present and so it was
considered to be an osteosarcoma. Radical radiotherapy was not
considered to be appropriate as these tumours are not radiosensitive. It
was decided to carry out immediate definitive surgery as this gave the
best chance of local control. The patient was fit for operation and there
was no obvious evidence of more widespread metastatic disease and so
further investigations were not arranged prior to surgery. A total
penectomy was carried out and the patient made a very satisfactory postoperative recovery. On follow up, he developed a meatal stenosis and has
required refashioning of the perineal urethrostomy.

Bone osteosarcoma has a reputation for being a very malignant
tumour which often metastasizes, most frequently to lung. Tumours
arising from soft tissue do not behave quite so aggressively, as illustrated
by this patient who was managed by radical surgery alone. As the tumour
was operable, prior chemotherapy was not necessary and there was no
value in its use adjuvantly.

He remains well and disease free six years later.

Case 4: Primary or metastatic?

A 77-year-old man was admitted with pain and discomfort from an ischaemic left foot. A left angioplasty was performed and the blood supply to his left leg markedly improved. However, during his admission, it transpired that he had a lesion on the penis for about 3 years, which had progressively increased in size. There was a polypoid lesion on the glans measuring 5 × 4 cm. The lesion was infiltrating down the shaft of the penis. There was ulceration and bleeding from the lesion.

How would you manage this patient?

This was a frail elderly gentleman with coexisting medical disease, who was markedly anaemic from a haemorrhaging lesion of the glans penis. It was obviously malignant and there was inguinal lymphadenopathy. He was transfused and commenced on antibiotics but continued to bleed profusely from the glans. Clotting indices and platelets were checked and found to be normal.

What further management would you propose?

He required emergency surgery to control the haemorrhage on the penis. At operation it was clear that tumour extended up both corpora to the level of the pubic bone. On dissection it was possible to get above the tumour in the corpora and the urethra was dissected separately. The tumour was also within the urethra but it was possible to get above this level. A perineal urethrostomy was performed and amputation achieved.

Histology revealed a malignant melanoma showing widespread infiltration of the distal penis. The surface of the tumour was largely ulcerated. Adjacent to the ulcerated tumour, the skin showed superficial spreading melanoma, presumably from where the main polypoid tumour had arisen. Tumour infiltrated widely and was present in vascular spaces, the corpus and at the resection margin, although the skin and urethra were clear, (**Figure 4.4.1**).

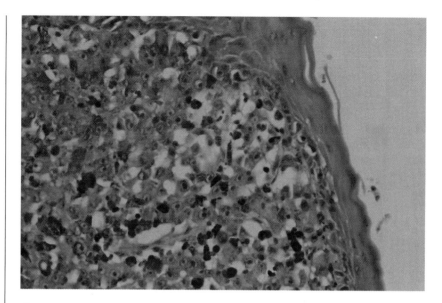

Figure 4.4.1 Malignant melanoma of the penis, H&E × 64

Further investigations revealed both hepatic and splenic metastases, (**Figure 4.4.2**).

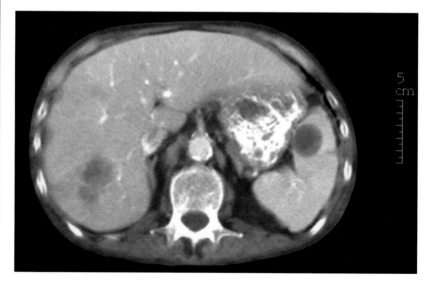

Figure 4.4.2 CT scan of abdomen

The patient is referred for further oncological management. What would you recommend?

The patient was an elderly frail gentleman who had widespread metastatic melanoma. It appeared to be arising from the penis although with such widespread disease, it could have been from another site. Melanoma is not a chemo-responsive tumour and as the patient was elderly, frail and had other medical conditions, it would not have been appropriate to give him chemotherapy.

Following surgery he made a good recovery. There was no indication for postoperative radiotherapy. The prognosis is obviously very poor.

SECTION 5: TESTIS

Case 1   The common testicular tumour   121
Case 2   The unusual testicular tumour   123
Case 3   Testicular pain from a rare tumour   125
Case 4   The extra testicular tumour   127
Case 5   Metastatic teratoma at presentation   131
Case 6   Metastatic seminoma at presentation   135

Case 1: The common testicular tumour

A 28-year-old man presented with a 3 – 4 week history of noticing a hard mass in his left testis. He had no history of trauma. Clinical examination revealed a hard mass in the lower pole of the left testis and scrotal ultrasound strongly suggested a testicular tumour.

How would you manage this patient?

He was likely to have a malignant testicular tumour and required urgent further management. Preoperative tumour markers would have been a guide to further management and the risk of metastatic disease. The preoperative tumour markers in this case were normal as was a chest X-ray. A left orchidectomy was performed and the appearances were of a classical seminoma (**Figure 5.1.1**). There were large cells with vesicular nuclei, clear cytoplasm and a lymphoid infiltrate. The cells were placental alkaline phosphase (PLAP) positive. A CT scan of the chest, abdomen and pelvis showed no evidence of nodal involvement or distant metastatic disease.

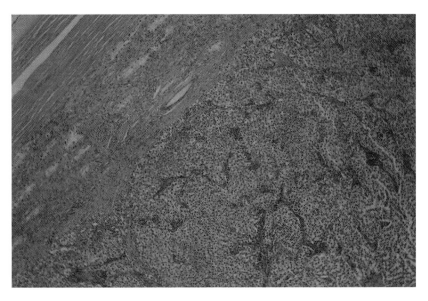

Figure 5.1.1   Seminoma of the testis, H&E × 12.8

Would you recommend any further treatment?

He had marker-negative stage 1 classical seminoma and the risk of recurrence without adjuvant radiotherapy is of the order of 20%. Therefore, he agreed to have a course of para-aortic radiotherapy as adjuvant treatment. A dose of 30 Gy in 15 fractions using parallel-opposed fields is the dose most widely used in the UK. There is evidence now that this can be reduced further to 20 Gy. Whilst awaiting radiotherapy treatment, arrangements were made for sperm analysis and sperm banking. The dose to the right testis was low and TLD (thermoluminescent dosimetry) measurements were made for documentation at the start of the course of radiotherapy.

An alternative adjuvant treatment would have been a course of Carboplatin chemotherapy (as in the TE19 study).

The prognosis is excellent.

Case 2: The unusual testicular tumour

A 76-year-old retired newspaper office worker initially presented with obstructive bladder symptoms. He was treated with an α-blocker but failed to show any improvement. At review, it was decided to admit him for TURP. In fact, he also had a testicular swelling which had been present for five months but he had ignored it. The mass was confirmed by ultrasonography and had the appearance of a possible malignancy. Preoperative tumour markers were normal. A left orchidectomy was performed and revealed a spermatocytic seminoma (**Figure 5.2.1**).

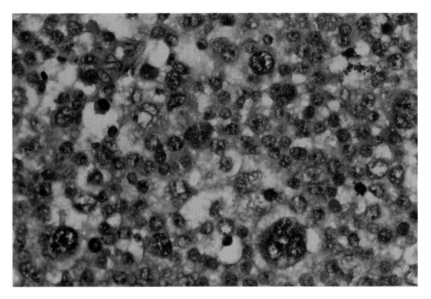

Figure 5.2.1   Typical spermatocytic seminoma, H&E × 128

What management would you recommend for this patient?

It is important in all patients with testicular masses to perform pre-operative tumour markers prior to orchidectomy. Spermatocytic seminoma is a very favourable pathological type and is associated with an excellent prognosis. Therefore, not surprisingly, the preoperative tumour markers were normal. Figure 5.2.1 shows typical appearances of a spermatocytic seminoma with sheets of cells showing moderate nuclear pleomorphism with a stipled chromatin pattern. Some cells have one or more small nucleoli. Occasional cells show a prominent central nucleolus. Cells have indistinct cytoplasm and some multinucleate tumour cells are present, staining positively for HCG. There is focal oedema within the tumour. The sheets of tumour cells are divided by occasional fibrous septa.

Baseline CT scan of the chest, abdomen and pelvis was carried out, although this was probably not entirely necessary. As expected, there were no signs of metastatic disease. No adjuvant therapy was given, or necessary, because of the non-aggressive nature of spermatocytic semi-noma. The patient has been followed up in the urology clinic because of obstructive symptoms but, as expected, over two years there has been no evidence of recurrence of the testicular tumour.

Case 3: Testicular pain from a rare tumour

A 39-year-old man presented with a six-month history of an inter-mittent painful testis. Clinical examination was entirely satisfactory. Testicular ultrasound showed a 5 × 2 × 3 mm echo free area in the left testis. Tumour markers were normal. He was considered to have an incidental benign cyst. Follow-up was arranged and a subsequent scan showed no change. He then complained of pain in the right groin and was tender at the head of the right epididymis. Tumour markers remained normal but ultrasound on this occasion showed a new lesion in the right testis of low echogenicity and not previously seen, which was solid.

How would you manage this patient?

He could have been managed with a follow-up scan to see whether the new area increased in size. It was reassuring that his tumour markers were negative. However, this new lesion was solid and really there was no option but to recommend a right inguinal orchidectomy. This was carried out. The small white nodule of tumour (**Figure 5.3.1**) measured 4 mm and was close to the rete testis. There was no tumour in the spermatic cord.

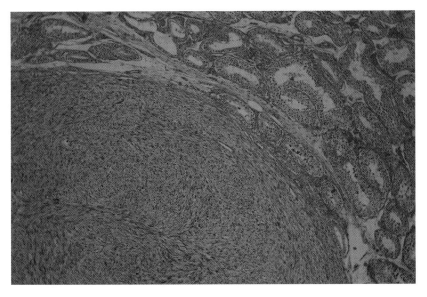

Figure 5.3.1   Small nodule in testis, H&E × 12.8

Pathology revealed a lesion consisting of fascicles of spindle shaped cells with blunt ended nuclei and numerous mitotic figures (**Figure 5.3.2**). The desmin and smooth muscle actin were positive. This was a leiomyosarcoma.

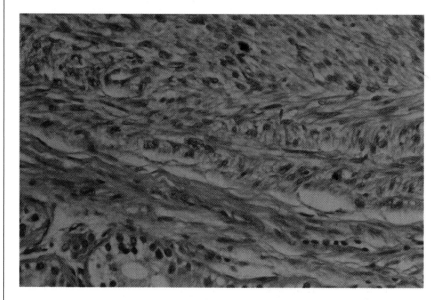

Figure 5.3.2   Pleomorphic spindle cells with mitoses, H&E × 64

What further management would you recommend?

A specialist in sarcoma pathology reviewed the pathology and he agreed with the diagnosis. He confirmed that the lesion would have been impalpable and was unlikely to have presented because of pain. The lesion appeared to be a primary, although it could have metastasised from elsewhere. No other findings were found on clinical examination. A CT scan of chest, abdomen and pelvis was carried out and this was entirely normal.

It was therefore decided to manage the patient with observation alone, following complete surgical excision. There is no evidence of the value of adjuvant chemotherapy in sarcomas in general and it would not be appropriate to give postoperative radiotherapy in this situation.

After over two years of follow up, there is no evidence of recurrence.

Case 4: The extra testicular tumour

A 28-year-old labourer suffered a football injury a year ago with swelling of the testicle. This resolved, but two or three months later, he noticed swelling of the right testis and a slight mucoid meatal discharge. The GP thought he had a suspiciously hard and enlarged right testis.

How would you advise this patient?

It was likely that this patient had a testicular tumour and he therefore needed immediate investigation. In fact, when seen by the urologist, the swelling was adjacent to the testicle and difficult to determine. Most of the testicle felt normal. Tumour markers for AFP and HCG were normal. Scrotal ultrasound was carried out (**Figure 5.4.1**). Chest X-ray was normal.

What does the ultrasound show?

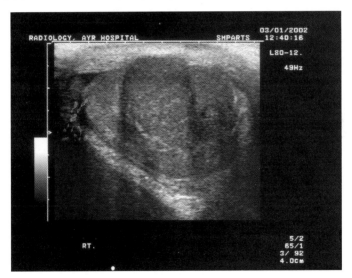

Figure 5.4.1   Ultrasound of right testis

How would you further manage this patient?

Scrotal ultrasonography showed a $30 \times 24 \times 20$ mm mass arising within the right testis. It was almost entirely solid and of a relatively uniform echogenic texture. Appearances were in keeping with a right testicular neoplasm. A right inguinal orchidectomy was carried out.

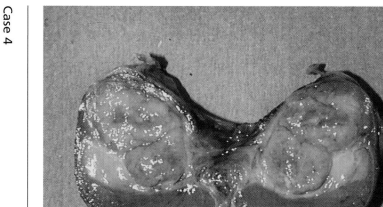

Figure 5.4.2   Macro of bivalved testis showing MTU (Malignant Teratoma Undifferentiated – light brown) and seminoma (white nodule)

What does the pathology show?

There was a soft grey-brown mass with a glistening grey area of scarred testis, (**Figure 5.4.2**). Most of the tumour is extratesticular, although a small area of typical seminoma was noted around the tubules within the testis itself. The tumour appeared to extend predominately from the rete testis into extra testicular tissue. The tumour had a striking appearance of islands of tumour cells with central necrosis interspersed with fibrous stroma. The nuclei were large and vesicular but were very pleomorphic with a high mitotic rate (26 per 10 HPF) (**Figure 5.4.3**). Immunohistochemistry showed the tumour cells to be positive for placental alkaline phosphatase and negative for HCG and AFP. There appeared to be some vascular invasion.

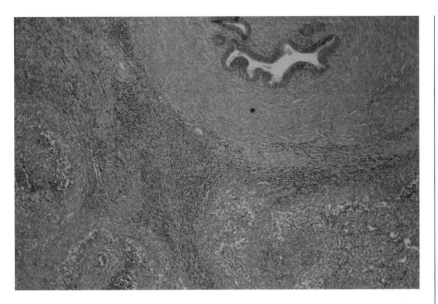

Figure 5.4.3 Extratesticular extension with tumour around the vas deferens, H&E × 64

It is extremely rare for testicular tumours to present as extra testicular masses. When there is induration or thickening of the epididymis, it is worth undertaking an ultrasound scan to check both that there is no abnormality and to assess the echotexture of the underlying testis. Further staging investigations included a CT scan of the chest, abdomen and pelvis, which did not show any evidence of metastatic disease.

This case illustrates that on clinical examination it would be quite easy to interpret, as was initially the case for some time, the lesion to be a chronic epididymitis. This substantially delayed the referral from the General Practitioner and emphasises the importance of radiological investigation if there is any concern about the nature of the scrotal swelling.

Does this patient require further treatment?

Although there was no evidence of metastatic disease and tumour markers were normal, this patient did have high-risk disease with pathology reporting malignant teratoma undifferentiated and considerable extra testicular disease. There was also vascular invasion. He was therefore given two courses of adjuvant chemotherapy using BEP. Prior to commencing chemotherapy, sperm analysis and storage was arranged.

The prognosis is excellent with an over 90% cure rate.

Case 5: Metastatic teratoma at presentation

A 19-year-old baker attended with both of his parents. He had more than a year long history of noticing a lump in the left testis which slowly increased in size. It was associated with a dull ache. There was no history of trauma and he felt well. He had no other complaints. His mother said he had a history of undescended testis when he was a child although this did not require surgical correction. On examination, there was a hard 2 cm craggy mass arising from the upper pole of the left testis. There was no inguinal lymphadenopathy. Preoperative tumour markers revealed a HCG of 4 and AFP of 53. A 19 mm, well defined, round hypoechoic mass arising from the upper pole of the testis was demonstrated on ultrasonography (**Figure 5.5.1**). A left orchidectomy was performed. Sperm analysis and storage were carried out.

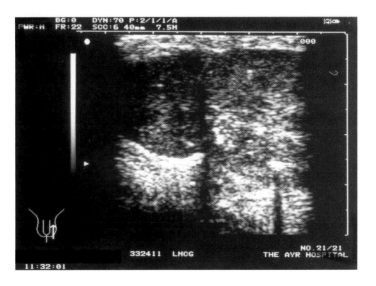

Figure 5.5.1 Ultrasound of testis

Staging investigations included a CT scan of chest, abdomen and pelvis. What does the abdominal CT scan show? (Figure 5.5.2)

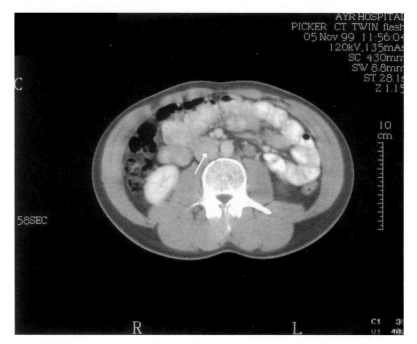

AYR HOSPITAL
PICKER CT TWIN flash
05 Nov 99 11:56:04
120kV,135mAs
SC 430mm
SW 8.8mm
ST 28.1s
Z 1.15

10
cm

C

58SEC

R   L

C1   3
U1   40

Figure 5.5.2   Abdominal CT scan

The patient obviously had a malignant tumour and the pre-operative tumour markers were in keeping with a teratoma. Histology confirmed a 25 mm testicular tumour invading the rete testis and epididymis, (**Figure 5.5.3**). The teratomatous component was papillary in areas and there were sheets of undifferentiated cells as well as more typical cartilage and glandular tissue with stromal areas. There was an extra testicular component, which was a seminoma. There was vascular invasion but the cord was not involved. Yolk sac tumour elements were also present. This was therefore a combined seminoma and teratoma with areas of embryonal carcinoma. The CT scan showed moderate left sided para-aortic lymphadenopathy. He had stage IIA disease.

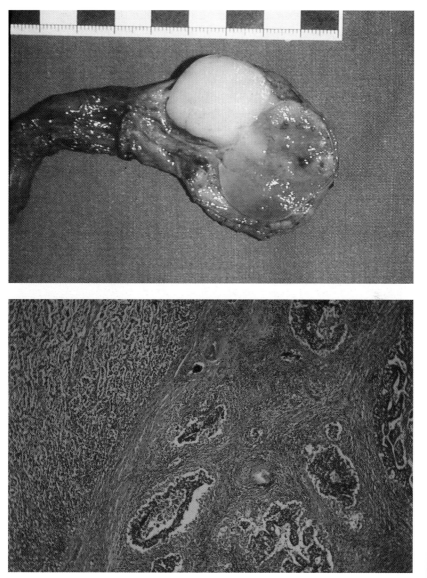

Figure 5.5.3 a Macro: Mixed tumour with partly cystic teratoma and a solid area of seminoma; **b** Mixed seminoma (upper left) and teratoma (lower right), H&E × 12.8

What treatment plan would you propose for this patient?

The plan of action was to give him three courses of BEP chemotherapy (Bleomycin, Etoposide and Cisplatin) and monitor the response with tumour markers. After two courses, the tumour markers were normal. After three courses, a post-treatment CT scan was carried out which showed a good response to chemotherapy but a residual para–aortic mass up to 2 cm in diameter.

What treatment recommendations would you make?

As he had residual retroperitoneal nodal disease evident on post-treatment CT scan, excision of the retroperitoneal tumour was carried out at laparotomy. The tumour consisted of three round masses in the retroperitoneal tissues, which were completely excised. Histology revealed mature teratoma with a small focus of immature stroma containing teratoma intermediate. There were no undifferentiated elements identified.

Should any further treatment be given?

The patient has had a good response to chemotherapy, confirmed both by imaging and surgical resection. This showed almost completely mature teratoma apart from one small focus. He did not require further chemotherapy, but needed to be followed up with regular tumour markers and CT scans.

Two years following his last surgery he remains very well and disease free.

Case 6: Metastatic seminoma at presentation

A 46-year-old man noticed swelling of the left testis over the last six months. He was well and had no pain or history of trauma. Clinical examination revealed a large swollen left testis. Scrotal ultrasound revealed a large (7 cm) heterogenous mass involving the left testis and suggestive of a testicular tumour. HCG was 186 and AFP 5. A left inguinal orchidectomy was performed. Histology revealed a classical seminoma with permeation of lymphatic channels at the edge of the tumour and just beneath the capsule (**Figure 5.6.1**). In addition, there was extensive vascular permeation within the cord.

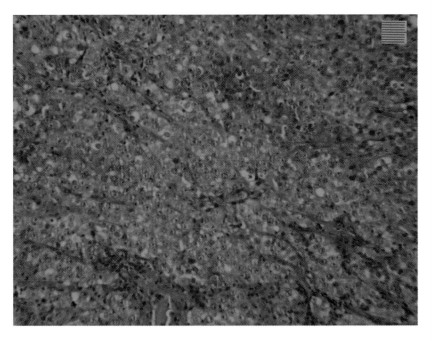

Figure 5.6.1 Typical seminoma with vesicular nuclei and prominent nucleoli (scale 0.1 mm).

Discuss his further management

In view of the size of tumour and the raised pre-operative tumour markers, he was at considerable risk of metastatic disease. A CT scan showed a large lobulated homogenous soft tissue mass extending from the left renal vein along the left para-aortic region to the bifurcation, measuring $9 \times 5 \times 4$ cm. There was no mediastinal lymphadenopathy.

Postoperatively, the tumour markers (HCG) rapidly fell to within normal range.

He had stage IIC disease and therefore required chemotherapy. He received treatment with Etoposide and Cisplatin. His renal function was satisfactory despite the considerable para-aortic disease. After four courses of chemotherapy, a further CT scan was performed which showed a reduction in the para-aortic lymphadenopathy from 9 cm to 2 cm.

What further management would you propose?

With such an excellent response, it was reasonable to put him on a surveillance programme. Surgery for the very small residual mass was probably not necessary but he required careful follow-up.

Five years after completing chemotherapy, he remains well with no evidence of recurrence. Serial CT scans have shown no change in the appearance of the small residual para-aortic mass.

APPENDICES

Appendix I   – Selected trials   139
Appendix II   – Drugs used in urological cancer treatment   141
Appendix III – Hormone therapy guideline for prostate cancer   143
Appendix IV   – PSA   145
Appendix V   – TNM staging   147
Appendix VI   – Gleason score   149
Appendix VII – Recommended reading   151

Trial	Site	Date/Status	Organisation
BS06 Radiotherapy *vs* observation Intravesical CT *vs* radiotherapy	Bladder	1991 → open	MRC CTU London NW1 2DA
BC2001 Standard RT *vs* Reduced volume RT ± chemotherapy	Bladder	2001 → open	Clinical Trials & Statistics Unit, The Institute of Cancer Research, (CTSU) Sutton, Surrey, SM2 5NG
RE04 Interferon α *vs* Interferon α + Interleukin 2 +5FU	Renal (metastatic)	2001 → open	MRC CTU
EORTC 30955 (Adjuvant IFNα, IL2 & 5FU)	Renal (high risk patients)	Open	EORTC Brussels, Belgium
TE18 Radiotherapy 30Gy *vs* 20Gy	Testis – Seminoma	Closed	MRC CTU
TE19 Carboplatin *vs* RT	Testis – Seminoma	Closed 2001	MRC CTU
TE08 Follow up CT scans 2 years *vs* 5 years	Testis	1998 → open	MRC CTU
PR07 Hormone therapy *vs* hormone therapy + Radiotherapy	Prostate	1999 → open	MRC CTU
Intercontinental prostate trial Post RT, rising PSA Intermittent *vs* continuous hormones	Prostate	Open 2002	CTSU
HDR brachytherapy boost trial	Prostate	Open	Mount Vernon Hospital
RTOG P.0011 Post prostatectomy study (rising PSA) RT *vs* hormones *vs* RT + hormones	Prostate	Open	CTSU
Intergroup RP56976V–327 Taxotere + Pred q 1/52 *vs* Taxotere + Pred q 3/52 *vs* Mitoxantrone + Pred q 3/52	Prostate (metastatic)	Closed 2002	
Intergroup S9916–329 Taxotere + Estramustine *vs* Mitoxantrone + Estramustine	Prostate (metastatic)	Closed 2002	

Appendix II: Drugs Used in Urological Cancer Treatment (including hormonal treatments)

KIDNEY

Aldesleukin (recombinant Interleukin 2) *(+/– lymphokine activated killer cells)*
Interferon Alfa – Interferon Alfa 2a (rbe) = Roferon A

Cytotoxics	Bleomycin, Dacarbazine, Floxurodine, Lomustine, Vinblastine, Vincristine
Cytotoxic regimes	
AD	Doxorubicin, Dacarbazine
CAD	Cyclophosphamide, Doxorubicin, Dacarbazine
CY-VA-DIC	Cyclophosphamide, Vincristine, Doxorubicin, Dacarbazine
MAI	Mesna, Doxorubicin, Ifosfamide
MAID	Mesna, Doxorubicin, Ifosfamide, Dacarbazine, Ifosfamide, Etoposide

Hormones

Progesterones	Medroxyprogesterone Acetate, Megestrol Acetate
Oestrogen–receptor antagonist	Tamoxifen

BLADDER

Intravesical therapy	Thiotepa, Mitomycin, Doxorubicin BCG (Bacillus Calmette-Guerin)
Cytotoxics	Bleomycin, Cisplatin, Cyclophosphamide, Doxorubicin, Etoposide, Floxuridine, Fluorouracil, Methotrexate, Vinblastine, Vincristine
Cytotoxic regimes	
CISCA	Cisplatin, Cyclophosphamide, Doxorubicin
CMV	Cisplatin, Methotrexate, Vinblastine
MAC	Methotrexate, Doxorubicin, Cyclophosphamide (Cisplatin for failure)
M-VAC	Methotrexate, Vinblastine, Daunorubicin, Cisplatin (or M-VAC high dose)
M-VEC	Methotrexate, Epirubicin, Vinblastine, Cisplatin
MVNC	Methotrexate, Vinblastine, Mitoxantrone, Carboplatin

PROSTATE

Oestrogen	Diethyl Stilboestrol (Stilboestrol) – used infrequently
Anti-androgen	Bicalutamide, Cyproterone, Flutamide
5-α reductase inhibitor	Finasteride (early stage cancer – inhibits testosterone metabolism)
LHRH analog	Buserelin, Goserelin, Leuprorelin acetate, Triptorelin
Cytotoxics	Cisplatin, Cyclophosphamide, Doxorubicin, Fluorouracil, Floxuridine, Hydroxyurea, Methotrexate, Mitoxantrone, Paclitaxel, Docetaxel

CEE   Cisplatin, Epirubicin, Estramustine
CFM   Cyclophosphamide, Fluorouracil, Megestrol
DS   Doxorubicin, Stilboestrol
Estramustine
Taxotere and Dexamethasone
Mitozantrone and Prednisolone

TESTICULAR
Cytotoxics   Carboplatin, Chlorambucil, Cyclophosphamide,
                                         Dactinomycin, Doxorubicin, Methotrexate

Combination chemotherapy
BEP   Cisplatin, Etoposide, Bleomycin or Ifosfamide
                                         Cisplatin, Ifosfamide, Etoposide or Vinblastine
CEB   Carboplatin, Etoposide, Bleomycin
HOP   Ifosfamide, Vincristine, Cisplatin
PVB   Etoposide, Vinblastine, Bleomycin
VAB VI   Vinblastine, Dactinomycin, Bleomycin,
                                         Cyclophosphamide, Cisplatin

Appendix III – Hormone Therapy Guideline for Prostate Cancer

Acute Hospitals NHS Trust
The Ayr Hospital

Local Guideline for the Management of Prostatic Cancer
Medical Hormonal control of Prostate Cancer

Day 1
Check U&E, LFT levels before starting treatment
Start antiandrogen
Cyproterone 100mg (Cyprostat®) Three times daily
Steroidal anti-androgen blocks Dihydrotestosterone at receptor and suppresses gonadotropins lowering testosterone plasma levels.

Between Day 4 and 7 (Cyproterone treatment ideally one week before and maximum of 3 weeks after LHRH injection)
Give Gonadorelin (LHRH) analogue – *ONE DOSE ONLY*
Goserelin acetate 3.6mg (Zoladex®) every 28 days or Leuprorelin acetate 3.75mg (Prostap SR®) monthly injection
Around 21 days from first injection testosterone castration levels are reached. Maintain by repeat depot injections at appropriate time intervals.

In some patients the 12 weekly or 3 monthly slow release preparation will be recommended by the Consultant Urologist
Goserelin 10.8mg (Zoladex® LA) or Leuprorelin acetate 11.25mg (Prostap® 3)
STOP Anti-androgen, 21 days after Gonadorelin (LHRH) analogue treatment
Repeat Gonadorelin (LHRH) analogue injection at recommended interval

---

If patient cannot use Cyproterone, a non steroidal anti-androgen may be considered

Summary recommendations prepared with reference to the COIN Guideline on Prostatic Cancer
An anti-androgen should be given before the FIRST Gonadorelin (LHRH) analogue depot injection to prevent the resulting increase in testosterone levels causing prostatic tumour growth and further complications. (Note an initial rise in testosterone levels may be seen with non-steroidal antiandrogens)

In the absence of anti-androgen therapy, on giving the first Gonadorelin analogue injection, testosterone levels will rise over the first two weeks increasing prostatic tumour growth and may cause spinal compression or ureteric obstruction. This applies to the first injection only, so antiandrogen therapy can be stopped three weeks after first injection given. Gonadorelin analogues are as effective as surgery with the same side effects but testosterone levels will increase if Gonadorelin analogue is stopped.

LHRH analogue if tolerated must be repeated according to the product recommendations.
Every 28 days if Goserelin or monthly if given Leuprorelin
Once tolerated consideration can be given to the use of a preparation lasting 3 months.
Goserelin 10.8mg (Zoladex LA™) – 12 weekly
Leuprorelin 11.25mg (Prostap 3™) – 3 monthly

Caution/Contraindication for the recommended groups of medicines:
If patient has an allergy to any of the above medicines or components of the medicines they should not be given.
Anti-androgens must be used with care in patients with moderate to severe hepatic

impairment and withdrawn if severe hepatic impairment if severe hepatic changes occur.

CSM warnings regarding long term use of Cyproterone and hepatic impairment are well documented, so regular monitoring of LFT's (liver function tests) must be carried out if antiandrogen use continued. Data sheets for Bicalutaminde and Flutamide also recommend monitoring LFT's.

Patients at risk of spinal cord compression or ureteric obstruction given anti-androgen therapy as tabled above should be monitored carefully after Gonadorelin analogue inserted. If signs of ureteric obstruction (renal impairment) or spinal cord compression (can present as – gait disturbance, paraesthesia, limb weakness, alteration to bowel or bladder function, back pain) immediate referral to secondary/tertiary care for treatment is advised.

Side effects –

Anti-androgen – Hot flushes (occurs less frequently with cyproterone), pruritis, breast tenderness, gynaecomastia, diarrhoea, nausea, vomiting, asthenia, dry skin, hepatic changes (elevated cholestasis, transaminases, and jaundice), hepatic failure, angina, heart failure, conduction defects, arrhythmias, ECG changes, thrombocytopenia, thrombo-embolism in patients with a previous history, breathlessness, hypochromic anaemia, may affect control in diabetic patients, osteoporosis, reduced sperm count and ejaculate volume.

If patient experiences hot flushes after LHRH treatment, these can be controlled by cyproterone 50mg increasing to 150mg daily in divided doses after food. Regular moni-toring of hepatic function must be carried out. Patients on warfarin should have INR checked regularly.

Bicalutamide must not be used in patients on astemizole, use cautiously in patients on cyclosporin or calcium channel blockers as dose reduction of these drugs may be required. Bicalutamide side effects may be increased with medicines, which inhibit drug oxidation (cimetidine, ketoconazole).

LHRH analogue – Hot flushes, decrease in libido, breast swelling and tenderness, temporary increase in bone pain, ureteric obstruction, spinal cord compression, loss of bone mineral density, arthralgia, skin rashes, local reactions at injection site including bruising, hypotension or hypertension may require treatment to be withdrawn. Rarely anaphylaxis.

Combination of anti-androgen and LHRH – heart failure, anorexia, dry mouth, dyspepsia, constipation, flatulence, dizziness, insomnia, somnolence, decreases libido, dyspnoea, impotence, nocturia, anaemia, alopecia, rash, sweating, hirsuitism, diabetes mellitus, hyperglycaemia, oedema, weight gain, weight loss, abdominal pain, chest pain, headache, pain, pelvic pain, chills.

The above information provides a summary for Hormonal manipulation of prostatic cancer only. Further information on each of the medicines listed can be found in the individual products current Summary of Product Characteristics.

The above guideline can be used in conjunction with the existing shared-care docu-ments for Zoladex and Prostap available from Medicines Information at the Ayr Hospital.

Appendix IV – PSA – Patient Information Sheet

The local guidelines on PSA for Primary Health Care and other practitioners in the acute sector

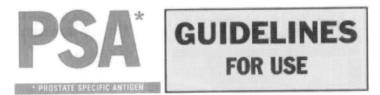

PSA* GUIDELINES FOR USE
* PROSTATE SPECIFIC ANTIGEN

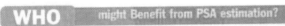

WHO might Benefit from PSA estimation?

● MEN OVER 45 YEARS ATTENDING A WELL MAN CLINIC.
(Generally not helpful in asymptomatic males over 70 years)

● MEN WITH LOWER URINARY TRACT SYMPTOMS COMPATIBLE WITH BLADDER OUTFLOW OBSTRUCTION (Prostatism)

● MEN WITH UNEXPLAINED
- WEIGHT LOSS
- ANAEMIA
- LOWER BACK PAIN

WHAT do the levels mean?

● PSA INCREASES WITH AGE. SO A VALUE WHICH IS SIGNIFICANT AT 40 YEARS MAY NOT BE AT 70 YEARS (SEE GRAPH).

● PSA IS NOT A DIAGNOSTIC TEST FOR PROSTATE CARCINOMA. THE HIGHER THE PSA VALUE, THE GREATER THE **RISK.**

● PSA VALUES WITHIN THE REFERENCE RANGE FOR AGE **DOES NOT EXCLUDE** PROSTATE CARCINOMA.

● PSA VALUES GREATER THAN THE REFERENCE RANGE ARE NOT DIAGNOSTIC FOR PROSTATE CARCINOMA. THEY MAY ALSO BE DUE TO:

- BENIGN PROSTATIC HYPERTROPHY
- PROSTATITIS.

● VERY HIGH LEVELS (>100ug/l) ARE GENERALLY DUE TO PROSTATE CARCINOMA.

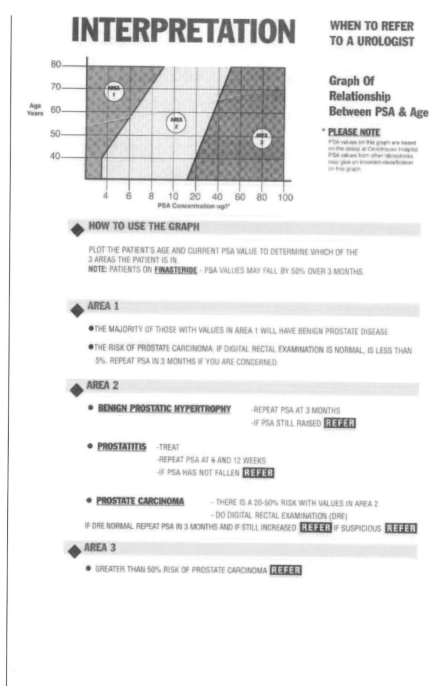

INTERPRETATION

WHEN TO REFER TO A UROLOGIST

Graph Of Relationship Between PSA & Age

* **PLEASE NOTE**
PSA values on this graph are based on the assay at Crosshouse Hospital. PSA values from other laboratories may give an incorrect classification on this graph.

◆ **HOW TO USE THE GRAPH**

PLOT THE PATIENT'S AGE AND CURRENT PSA VALUE TO DETERMINE WHICH OF THE 3 AREAS THE PATIENT IS IN.
NOTE: PATIENTS ON **FINASTERIDE** - PSA VALUES MAY FALL BY 50% OVER 3 MONTHS.

◆ **AREA 1**

● THE MAJORITY OF THOSE WITH VALUES IN AREA 1 WILL HAVE BENIGN PROSTATE DISEASE

● THE RISK OF PROSTATE CARCINOMA, IF DIGITAL RECTAL EXAMINATION IS NORMAL, IS LESS THAN 5%. REPEAT PSA IN 3 MONTHS IF YOU ARE CONCERNED.

◆ **AREA 2**

● **BENIGN PROSTATIC HYPERTROPHY**   -REPEAT PSA AT 3 MONTHS
                                      -IF PSA STILL RAISED **REFER**

● **PROSTATITIS**   -TREAT
                    -REPEAT PSA AT 6 AND 12 WEEKS
                    -IF PSA HAS NOT FALLEN **REFER**

● **PROSTATE CARCINOMA**   - THERE IS A 20-50% RISK WITH VALUES IN AREA 2
                           - DO DIGITAL RECTAL EXAMINATION (DRE)
IF DRE NORMAL REPEAT PSA IN 3 MONTHS AND IF STILL INCREASED **REFER** IF SUSPICIOUS **REFER**

◆ **AREA 3**

● GREATER THAN 50% RISK OF PROSTATE CARCINOMA **REFER**

URINARY BLADDER

Ta		Noninvasive papillary
Tis		*In situ*: 'flat tumour'
T1		Subepithelial connective tissue
T2		Muscularis
	T2a	Inner half
	T2b	Outer half
T3		Beyond muscularis
	T3a	Microscopically
	T3b	Extravesical mass
T4		
	T4a	Prostate, uterus, vagina
	T4b	Pelvic wall, abdominal wall
N0		No node involvement
N1		Single <2 cm
N2		Single >2 to 5 cm, multiple <5 cm
N3		>5 cm
M0		No distant metastasis
M1		Distant metastasis

KIDNEY

T1	≤7.0 cm; limited to the kidney
T2	>7.0 cm; limited to the kidney
T3	Into major veins; adrenal or perinephric invasion
T4	Invades beyond Gerota fascia
N0	No node involvement
N1	Single regional lymph node
N2	More than one regional lymph node
M0	No distant metastasis
M1	Distant metastasis

RENAL PELVIS, URETER

Ta	Noninvasive papillary
Tis	*In situ*
T1	Subepithelial connective tissue
T2	Muscularis
T3	Beyond muscularis
T4	Adjacent organs, perinephric fat
N0	No node involvement
N1	Single ≤2 cm
N2	Single > 2 to 5 cm, multiple ≤ 5 cm
N3	> 5 cm
M0	No distant metastasis
M1	Distant metastasis

TESTIS

pTis	Intratubular
pT1	Testis and epididymis, no vascular/lymphatic invasion
pT2	Testis and epididymis with vascular/lymphatic invasion or tunica vaginalis
pT3	Spermatic cord
pT4	Scrotum
N0	No node involvement
N1	≤2 cm
N2	>2 to 5 cm
N3	>5 cm
M0	No metastasis
M1a	Non-regional lymph node or pulmonary metastasis
M1b	Non-pulmonary visceral metastasis

PROSTATE

T1		Not palpable or visible
	T1a	≤5%
	T1b	>5%
	T1c	Needle biopsy
T2		Confined within prostate
	T2a	One lobe
	T2b	Both lobes
T3		Through prostatic capsule
	T3a	Extracapsular
	T3b	Seminal vesicles(s)
T4		Fixed or invades adjacent structures: bladder neck, external sphincter, rectum, levator muscles, pelvic wall
N0		No node involvement
N1		Regional lymph node(s)
M0		No metastasis
M1a		Non-regional lymph node(s)
M1b		Bone(s)
M1c		Other site(s)

PENIS

Tis	*In situ*
Ta	Noninvasive verrucous carcinoma
T1	Subepithelial connective tissue
T2	Corpus spongiosum, cavernosum
T3	Urethra, prostate
T4	Other adjacent structures
N0	No node involvement
N1	One superficial inguinal node
N2	Multiple or bilateral superficial inguinal nodes
N3	Deep inguinal or pelvic nodes
M0	No distant metastasis
M1	Distant metastasis

Appendix VI – Gleason Score

The biological behaviour of prostate cancer is correlated to its histological appearance. Several scoring systems of the classification of grade have been developed, but the Gleason score is the most popular. It is based on the extent to which the tumour cells are arranged into recognisably glandular structures. Gleason described it in 1966. It categorises the appearance into five groups, scoring 1 to 5. The system takes into account that the microscopic appearances of any one tumour vary. The final score is the sum of the two most differing appearances in terms of area, (e.g. Gleason 4+3). If there is a single pattern, then this score is doubled. Therefore the score is in the range 2–10. It is sometimes referred to as the double Gleason score.

Grade 1 – very well differentiated adenocarcinoma, forming almost normal glands appearing as very well defined clumps.

Grade 2 – well differentiated adenocarcinoma, which is slightly less uniform, separated by more abundant stroma. Clumps of tumour cells are slightly less well defined.

Grade 3 – moderately differentiated adenocarcinoma, with polymorphic glands. There are abundant stroma and poorly defined clumps of tumour cells.

Grade 4 – poorly differentiated carcinoma, with poorly defined and differentiated clumps containing poorly structured and fused glands.

Grade 5 – sheets of undifferentiated tumour cells with minimal gland formation.

Appendix VII – Recommended reading

Comprehensive Textbook of Genitourinary Oncology, 2nd Edition
Nicholas J Vogelzang, Peter T Scardino, William U Shipley &
Donald S Coffey
Lippincott Williams & Wilkins, 2000

Renal, Bladder, Prostate and Testicular Cancer: An Update
Progress and Controversies in Oncological Urology VI (PACIOU VI)
Edited by Karl H Kurth, Gerald H J Mickisch & Fritz H Schroder
Parthenon Publishing, 2001

Improving Outcomes in Urological Cancers
National Institute for Clinical Excellence, September 2002

International Handbook of Prostate Cancer
Edited by David Kirk
Euromed Communications Ltd, 1999

Textbook of Prostate Cancer – Pathology, Diagnosis and Treatment
Amir V Kaisary, Gerald P Murphy, Louis Denis & Keith Griffiths
Martin Dunitz Ltd, 1999

Prostate Cancer, 2nd Edition
Roger S Kirby, Timothy J Christmas & Michael K Brawer
Mosby International Ltd, 2001

Renal Cell Carcinoma: Molecular Biology, Immunology and Clinical
Management
Edited by Ronald M Bukowski & Andrew Novick
Humana Press, 2000

Classic Papers in Urology I–III
(Pages 45–133)
Edited by E W Gerharz, M Emberton & T O'Brien
Isis Medical Media, 1999

A W Partin et al
JAMA 1997; 227: 1445–51

J E Oesterling, S K Martin, E J Bergstraich, F C Lowe
The use of PSA in staging patients with newly diagnosed prostate
cancer
JAMA 1993; 2269(1): 57–60

J E Oesterling
Using PSA to eliminate the staging radionuclide bone scan
Urol Clin North Am 1993; 20: 705–711

Index

General Index	Page Number
Abdominal pain	73–75
Adjuvant chemotherapy, testicular tumours	122, 129
Adjuvant radiotherapy, stage I seminoma	122
Alphafetoprotein (AFP), testicular tumours	132
Aneurysm, kidney	74
Angiomyelolipoma, kidney	73–75
Anti-androgen therapy	143–144
Asbestos-related lung disease	14
BCG therapy, carcinoma of bladder	3–5, 10, 15, 19
BEP (bleomycin, etoposide and cisplatin) chemotherapy, mixed testicular tumour	133
Bicalutamide	56, 144
Biopsy	
liver metastases	62–63
prostate	27
in situ . . . . . . ¿ carcinoma	4
Bladder carcinoma	1–24
advanced	21–24
chemosensitive	17–19
grade III	7–8, 17–19
multiple	9–11
prostate carcinoma with	13–15, 41–43
in situ	3–5
TNM staging	147
treatment drugs	141
upper urinary tract surveillance	85–89
Bleomycin, BEP chemotherapy, mixed testicular tumour	133
Bone marrow	
interferon	94–95
prostate carcinoma	65–69
Bone metastases, prostate carcinoma	35–36, 37–39, 41, 45–50, 55–58
Bone scintigraphy, prostate carcinoma	38–39, 67–68 (Fig.)
Brachytherapy, prostate carcinoma	36
Brain, angiomyelolipoma	74–75
Carboplatin, stage I seminoma	122
Casodex (bicalutamide)	56, 144
Chemotherapy	
bladder carcinoma	18

drugs	141–142
intravesical	9–10, 15
prostate carcinoma and	63
renal failure	21–24
testicular tumours	122, 129, 133, 136
Cisplatin	
BEP chemotherapy, mixed testicular tumour	133
metastatic seminoma	136
renal failure	23–24
Complex cyst, kidney	77–79
Computed tomography	
bladder carcinoma	8, 17–18, 22
complex renal cyst	77
lung metastases	102–103
perinephric haemorrhage	73–74
prostate carcinoma	45–46, 55–56, 65
renal carcinoma	81, 91, 93, 94
teratoma	132
Corticosteroids, optic nerve compression	57
Creatinine, bladder carcinoma	7–8
Cyproterone	38, 143, 144
Cyst (complex), kidney	77–79
Cystectomy	8, 10–11, 15
Cystoscopy	11
Dexamethasone	69
Disseminated intravascular coagulation	69
Efudex cream (5-fluorouracil)	110
Electron therapy, penis	111–112
Embolization (therapeutic), angiomyelolipoma of kidney	74, 75
Embryonal carcinoma	132
Epididymis	129
Erythrocyte sedimentation rate	98
Etoposide	
BEP chemotherapy, mixed testicular tumour	133
metastatic seminoma	136
Extratesticular seminoma	127–129, 132
Fibrous histiocytoma, rib	36
Fistula, urethro-rectal	32–34
5-fluorouracil (Efudex) cream	110
Flutamide, prostate carcinoma bone metastases	56
Foamy cells, papillary renal carcinoma	82 (Fig.)
Fracture, prostate carcinoma metastasis	49
Gastrointestinal haemorrhage	18–19

Gleason score, prostate carcinoma | 149
Gonadorelin (LHRH) therapy | 53–54, 143, 144
Goserelin (Zoladex) | 38, 53–54, 56, 143
Grafting, carcinoma of penis | 110
Granuloma, BCG therapy | 4

Haemorrhage
   malignant melanoma of penis | 114
   perinephric fat | 74
Histiocytoma, rib | 36
Hormonal therapy
   drugs | 141
   prostate carcinoma | 38, 43, 53–54, 143–144
   renal carcinoma metastases | 99
Hot flushes, 144
Human chorionic gonadotropin (HCG) | 132
Humerus, prostate carcinoma metastasis | 47–50
Hydronephrosis | 21–22

Ibuprofen | 69
Immunotherapy
   bladder carcinoma | 3–5
   renal carcinoma | 91–95
Infection, bladder carcinoma | 4
In situ carcinoma
   bladder | 3–5
   penis | 109–110
   see also Intraepithelial prostate carcinoma
Interferon, renal carcinoma | 93–95, 103–105
Intraepithelial prostate carcinoma | 28
Intravenous urography
   renal carcinoma | 97–98
   transitional cell carcinoma | 86 (Fig.)
Intravesical chemotherapy | 9–10, 15
Iodine brachytherapy, prostate carcinoma | 36

Kidney tumours | 71–105
   treatment drugs | 141

Laparoscopic radical prostatectomy | 31–32
Laser ablation, renal pelvis tumour | 11, 87
Left renal vein, seminoma extension | 135–136
Leiomyosarcoma, testis | 125–126
Leucopenia, interferon and | 94
Leuprorelin | 143
Liver, prostate carcinoma metastases | 61–63
Lung, renal carcinoma metastases | 98–99, 101–105

Luteinizing hormone-releasing hormone
    (LHRH) therapy   53–54, 143, 144
Lymphangiography, magnetic resonance   65
Lymph nodes
    bladder carcinoma   18, 23
    mixed testicular tumour   133–134
    prostate carcinoma   45, 65
    renal carcinoma   93, 99
Lymphoedema, prostate carcinoma   45

Magnetic resonance imaging
    lymphangiography   65
    prostate carcinoma   31, 37, 59, 60 (Fig.)
Malignant melanoma, penis   115–117
Masses, abdomen   73–75
Mediastinal lymph nodes, renal carcinoma   99
Medroxyprogesterone, renal carcinoma
    metastases   99
Melanoma, penis   115–117
Metastases
    malignant melanoma   116–117
    renal carcinoma   98–99, 101–105
    seminoma   135–136
    teratoma   131–134
    unknown primary   101–105
    see also Lymph nodes; Prostate carcinoma
Mixed testicular tumour   132–134
Multiple bladder carcinoma   9–11

Nephrectomy
    complex renal cyst   78–79
    renal carcinoma   98
    transitional cell carcinoma   87
Nephroma, cystic   78
Nephrostomy, ureteric catheter placement   33

Optic nerve compression, prostate carcinoma
    metastases   57
Orbit, prostate carcinoma metastases   56–58
Orthotopic reconstruction, radical cystectomy   15
Osteosarcoma, penis   113–114

Pain
    abdomen   73–75
    prostate carcinoma metastases   56
Palliative radiotherapy
    bladder carcinoma   18, 19
    prostate carcinoma metastases   56

Papillary carcinoma of bladder	9–11
Papillary renal carcinoma	81–83
Para-aortic adjuvant radiotherapy, stage I seminoma	122
Para-aortic lymph nodes, mixed testicular tumour	133–134
Patient information sheet, prostate-specific antigen	145–146
Penectomy	114, 115
Penis	107–117
carcinoma	109–110, 111–112, 148
malignant melanoma	115–117
osteosarcoma	113–114
prostate carcinoma metastasis	41–43
Perinephric fat, haemorrhage	74
Pleura	
asbestosis	14
malignant effusion	101–102
Preoperative tumour markers, testicular tumours	121, 123, 131–132, 135
Proptosis	57
Prostate carcinoma	25–69
bladder carcinoma with	13–15, 41–43
bone metastases	35–36, 37–39, 41, 45–50, 55–58
Gleason score	149
hormonal therapy	38, 43, 53–54, 143–144
liver metastases	61–63
orbital metastases	56–58
penis, metastases	41–43
spinal cord compression	51–54
strontium therapy	66
TNM staging	148
treatment drugs	141–142
Prostatectomy, radical	13–14, 31–32
Prostate-specific antigen	
bone scintigraphy	39
intraepithelial prostate carcinoma	28–29
patient information sheet	145–146
Prostatic acid phosphatase, prostate carcinoma metastasis	41–42
Prostatitis	27
PSA see Prostate-specific antigen	
Ptosis	57

Radionuclide scintigraphy, prostate
   carcinoma   38–39, 67–68 (Fig.)
Radiotherapy
   bladder carcinoma   8, 18, 19
   para–aortic adjuvant, stage I seminoma   122
   penis, carcinoma   111–112
   prostate carcinoma   46, 49, 53, 56, 57, 59,
        65–66

Rectum, fistula   32–34
Renal carcinoma
   histology   82 (Fig.), 92 (Fig.)
   immunotherapy   91–95
   metastases   98–99, 101–105
   papillary   81–83
   TNM staging   147
Renal failure   7–8, 21–24
Renal pelvis, transitional cell carcinoma   11, 85–89
Retroperitoneal adjuvant radiotherapy,
   stage I seminoma   122
Retroperitoneal metastases, mixed testicular
   tumour   133–134
Rib, prostate carcinoma metastasis   35–36

Sarcomas, leiomyosarcoma   125–126
Scrotum, radiotherapy to penile carcinoma   111
Seminoma   121–122
   extratesticular   127–129, 132
   metastases   135–136
   spermatocytic   123–124
Sinerem, magnetic resonance
   ymphangiography   65
Skin reaction, radiotherapy   111–112
Soft tissue osteosarcoma   113–114
Solitary bone metastasis, prostate carcinoma   45–50
Spermatocytic seminoma   123–124
Spinal cord compression, prostate carcinoma
   metastases   51–54
Squamous carcinoma *in situ*, penis   109–110
Strontium, prostate carcinoma metastases   56, 66
Surgery
   carcinoma of penis   110
   cystectomy   8, 10–11, 15
   malignant melanoma of penis   115–117
   prostatectomy   13–14, 31–32
   renal carcinoma metastases   99
   see also Nephrectomy
Surveillance, upper urinary tract, bladder
   carcinoma   85–89

Teratoma	128 (Fig.), 129, 132–134
Testis	
treatment drugs	142
tumours	119–136, 148
Thermoluminescent dosimetry, testis	122
Thrombocytopenia	
bone marrow infiltration	66, 68 (Fig.), 69
interferon	94–95
TNM staging	147–148
Transitional cell carcinoma	
renal pelvis	11, 85–89
TNM staging	147
see also Bladder carcinoma	
Transrectal ultrasound, prostate biopsy	27
Trials, cancer treatments	139
Tumour markers, testicular tumours	121, 123, 131–132, 135
Ultrasound	
liver metastases	61
prostate biopsy	27
testis	127, 131
Unknown primary, metastases	101–105
Upper urinary tract surveillance	85–89
Ureteric catheters	33
Ureteroscopy	11
Urethro-rectal fistula	32–34
Urinary diversion	33
Urothelium	5 (Fig.)
Vascular malformations	74–75
Vascular spread, seminoma	135–136
Vertebrae, prostate carcinoma metastases	52–53
Xanthoma, rib	36
Yolk sac tumour	132
Zoladex (goserelin)	38, 53–54, 56, 143